District Nursing
at a Glance

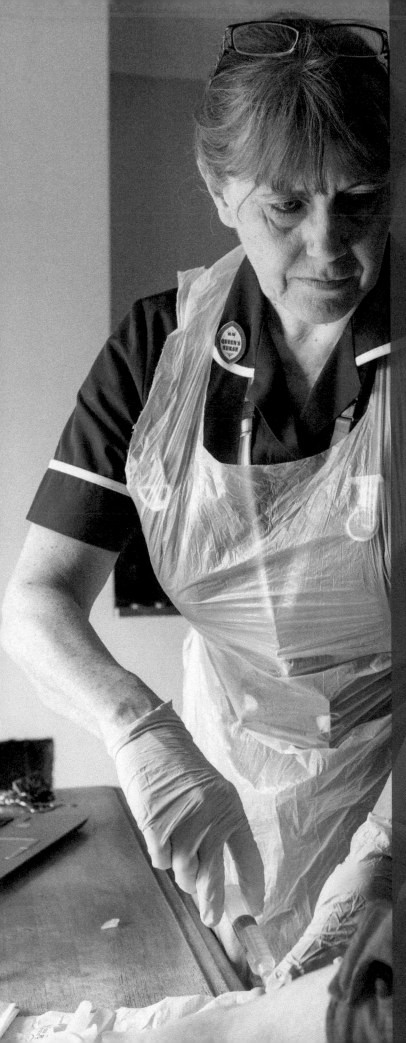

District
Nursing
at a Glance

Edited by

Matthew Bradby
The Queen's Nursing Institute
1A Henrietta Place
London, UK

WILEY Blackwell

This edition first published 2022
© 2022 John Wiley & Sons Ltd

The right of Matthew Bradby to be identified as the author of the editorial material in this work has been asserted in accordance with law.

Registered Offices
John Wiley & Sons, Inc., 111 River Street, Hoboken, NJ 07030, USA
John Wiley & Sons Ltd, The Atrium, Southern Gate, Chichester, West Sussex, PO19 8SQ, UK

Editorial Office
9600 Garsington Road, Oxford, OX4 2DQ, UK

For details of our global editorial offices, customer services, and more information about Wiley products, visit us at www.wiley.com.

Wiley also publishes its books in a variety of electronic formats and by print-on-demand. Some content that appears in standard print versions of this book may not be available in other formats.

Library of Congress Cataloging-in-Publication Data

Names: Bradby, Matthew, editor.
Title: District nursing at a glance / Matthew Bradby.
Other titles: At a glance series (Oxford, England)
Description: Hoboken, NJ: Wiley-Blackwell 2022. | Series: At a glance |
    Includes bibliographical references and index.
Identifiers: LCCN 2021028067 (print) | LCCN 2021028068 (ebook) |
    ISBN 9781119023418 (paperback) | ISBN 9781119023425 (adobe pdf) |
    ISBN 9781119023456 (epub)
Subjects: MESH: Community Health Nursing | United Kingdom
Classification: LCC RT98 (print) | LCC RT98 (ebook) | NLM WY 106 | DDC
    610.73/43–dc23
LC record available at https://lccn.loc.gov/2021028067
LC ebook record available at https://lccn.loc.gov/2021028068

Cover Design: Wiley
Cover Image: Courtesy of The Queen's Nursing Institute

Set in 9.5/11.5pt Minion Pro by Straive, Pondicherry, India
Printed and bound by CPI Group (UK) Ltd, Croydon, CR0 4YY

C9781119023418_230222

This book is dedicated to Alison Burton Shepherd, Queen's Nurse (1965–2020).

Contents

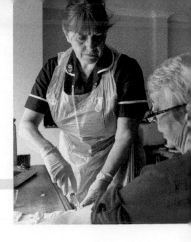

Part 4 Caring for the whole person in the community 43

Part 5 Physical and mental health in the community 87

Part 6 Specialisms in the community 139

Preface

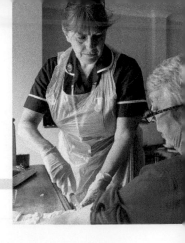

The nurses who have written the chapters of this book are Queen's Nurses. The title of Queen's Nurse was reintroduced by the Queen's Nursing Institute in 2007 as a way of recognising the excellence of community nursing practice in England, Wales and Northern Ireland, the three countries where the charity operates. The title has also subsequently been reintroduced north of the border by the Queen's Nursing Institute Scotland. Today there are over 1700 Queen's Nurses in every community specialism, not just district nursing.

This book is divided into six main parts, preceded by an introductory section.

Part 1 Introduction aims to give the reader an introduction to the heritage of the district nursing profession and also to the charity, the Queen's Nursing Institute, which has been indelibly associated with the profession for over 130 years.

Part 2 The learning environment gives the reader an introduction to the framework of district nurse education at the present time, although this framework continues to evolve and develop at a rapid pace.

Part 3 Working in the community focuses on the district nursing team, on the systems and ethics that guide its successful working, and on the place of the individual within that team.

Part 4 Caring for the whole person in the community looks at the people district nurses will meet in their professional life as they carry out visits in their local community. It looks at the whole person, as a member of a family, of a culture and a community. That person may have carers, who may be friends or family members, or support workers. We have tried to use the word 'person' rather than 'patient'; for people living with one or more long-term conditions; they may not view themselves as a patient when they are being cared for at home, but they are all people whose quality of life is made significantly better by the support of a district nurse. Often it is this support that enables the person to live at home and avoid admission to hospital or residential care; in this role the nurse is both a vital support to the individual and their family and also a hugely important part of the whole health and social care system.

Part 5 Physical and mental health in the community looks at a whole range of physical and mental health conditions that are commonly encountered by district nurses during the course of their work. The conditions covered in the book are not meant to be exhaustive but are indicative of the kind of long-term conditions that require an in-depth knowledge of the person and careful case management of their condition. The skilled district nurse will have the ability, working in partnership with the person she cares for, to progress and improve their health. He or she will also be one of the most important sources of emotional and psychological support to the person and their family.

Part 6 Specialisms in the community explores some of the other specialisms that district nurses will encounter during their work. Again, this is not meant to be an exhaustive list but an introduction to some of the other specialisms that are employed by healthcare providers and voluntary organisations. This links back to Part 3 and the importance of collaborative working, drawing on the skills of the most suitably qualified professionals to deliver enhanced care to people in need.

Additional sources of information

Some of the chapters contain links to additional sources of information and a final chapter gives a list of References and further reading.

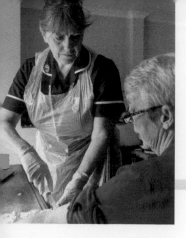

Acknowledgements

The editor would like to thank the staff of The Queen's Nursing Institute for their support and encouragement, in particular Dr Crystal Oldman CBE, Dr Agnes Fanning and Joanna Sagnella, QNI Publications Manager, who produced many of the illustrations in this book, and QNI interns Joanna Boughtflower, William Carter, Olivia Hicks, Alice Knapton and Chloe McCallum for their valuable assistance.

The editor would also like to thank Hallam Medical, Malinko, Kate Stanworth, Mark Hakansson, Harriet Stuart-Jones and the editorial staff at Wiley.

Queen's Nurses are supported by funding from the National Garden Scheme, a national charity that opens private gardens to raise money for nursing and caring charities. Since 1927 the garden scheme has raised millions of pounds for healthcare in the community.

Introduction to District Nursing

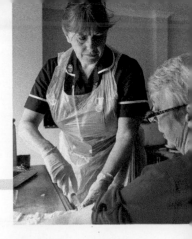

A District Nurse is a specialist generalist nurse in the community, an expert who is accountable at an advanced level of practice.

The District Nurse serves a whole community, holding and being responsible for a large and varied caseload of people with complex health needs, and managing admission to and discharge from that caseload. They are responsible for autonomous clinical decision-making, deploying a team of regulated and unregulated staff to deliver care in peoples' homes, and leading all the nursing care required. A community staff nurse is one of the nurses working under the direction of the District Nurse. District Nurses work above all in people's homes and may give support to staff working in Nursing and Residential Homes too.

A qualified District Nurse is prepared for their role with a post-registration Specialist Practitioner Qualification in District Nursing (SPQ DN) at a Higher Education Institution. These post-registration programmes are currently approved and regulated by the Nursing and Midwifery Council (NMC) to ensure consistency and quality of standards for education and practice and to prepare nurses for the role of an autonomous practitioner.

Specialist Practitioner Qualifications are also available in Community Children's Nursing (CCN), Community Learning Disabilities Nursing (CLDN), Community Mental Health Nursing (CMHN), and General Practice Nursing (GPN), and the NMC is consulting on additional qualifications for other community specialisms (2021).

This book describes some of the most important parts of a District Nurses' role. It is not intended as an exhaustive or comprehensive list of everything that a District Nurse might be called upon to do, which is always changing and developing. The Covid-19 pandemic has changed the landscape of nursing in the community profoundly and rapidly, and District Nurses are now caring for many people who are recovering from this novel disease.

The landscape of health services in the United Kingdom is also changing, and there is growing variation between England, Wales, Scotland, and Northern Ireland. Healthcare policy demands that more care is delivered in people's homes and communities and a greater reliance on self-care and the prevention of ill-health, lessening people's dependence on hospital services.

It is an exciting time to be a District Nurse, working with people, carers, and families across the life course, helping them to maintain health and independence, in communities in every part of the UK.

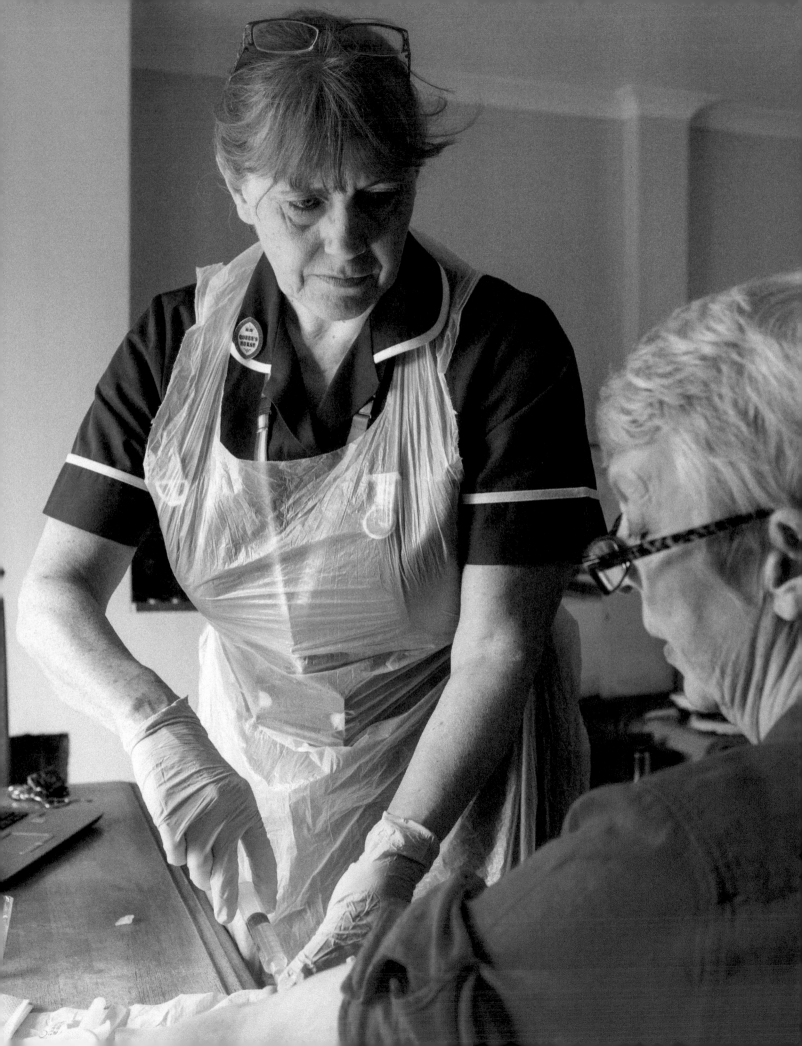

Introduction

Part 1

Chapters

1 The early history of district nursing

Matthew Bradby

Figure 1.1   Cartoon of Queen's Nurses in 1918.

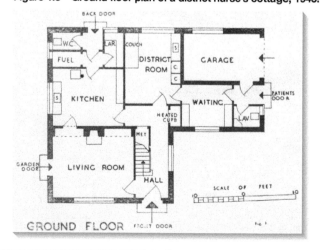

Figure 1.2   Queen's Nurse with a bicycle, c. 1900.

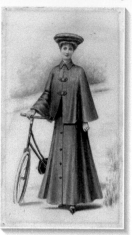

Figure 1.3   The celebrated midwife's case, 1925.

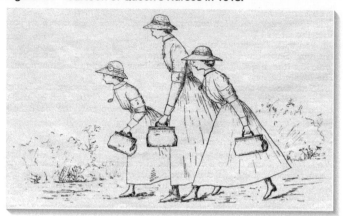

Figure 1.4   Queen's Nurses magazine advert, 1913.

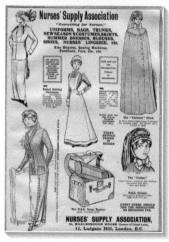

Figure 1.5   Ground floor plan of a district nurse's cottage, 1945.

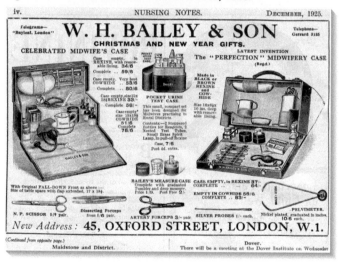

Figure 1.6   Architect's design for a district nurse's cottage, 1945.

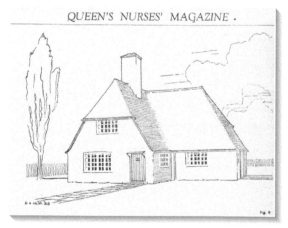

District Nursing at a Glance, First Edition. Edited by Matthew Bradby.
© 2022 John Wiley & Sons Ltd. Published 2022 by John Wiley & Sons Ltd.

The district nursing movement started in Victorian England in the mid nineteenth century. The Victorian period was characterised by rapidly growing cities, where many people lived in extremely poor, cramped conditions. Malnutrition and unclean water supplies contributed to severe and regular outbreaks of contagious diseases, such as cholera, typhus and tuberculosis, which were the mass killers of the period. District nursing as an organised movement began when William Rathbone (1819–1902), a wealthy Liverpool merchant and philanthropist, employed a nurse, Mary Robinson, to care for his wife at home during her final illness. In May 1859 William Rathbone's wife died, and he later wrote:

> it occurred to me to engage Mrs. Robinson, her nurse, to go into one of the poorest districts of Liverpool and try, in nursing the poor, to relieve suffering and to teach them the rules of health and comfort. I furnished her with the medical comforts necessary, but after a month's experience she came to me crying and said that she could not bear any longer the misery she saw. I asked her to continue the work until the end of her engagement with me (which was three months), and at the end of that time, she came back saying that the amount of misery she could relieve was so satisfactory that nothing would induce her to go back to private nursing, if I were willing to continue the work (Hardy, 1981).

William Rathbone decided to try to extend the service started with Mary Robinson, but soon found that there was a lack of trained nurses and that nurse training was disorganised and very variable in quality. In 1860, he wrote to Florence Nightingale, who advised him to create a nurse training school and home for nurses attached to the Liverpool Royal Infirmary and, with typical Victorian organisation and energy, this was built by May 1863.

For district nursing purposes, the city was divided into 18 'districts', each made up of a group of parishes. Each district was under the charge of a Lady Superintendent drawn from a wealthy family. The system was non-sectarian, though local ministers were encouraged to become involved. Liverpool was not alone in experiencing poverty and ill health and district nursing associations soon spread to other industrial cities – Manchester in 1864, Derby in 1865, Leicester in 1867, and London in 1868. The Victorian district nursing movement was characterised by several long running debates, which had their roots in views about social class and the role of working women. It took time, experimentation and organisation for the training of district nurses to become established. This coincided with an era of great advances in medical science and new ideas about the emancipation of women into paid occupations (Figures 1.1 and 1.2).

District nurses had to work hard to gain the confidence and trust of poorer families, for whom home nursing was a novelty: extended families were used to caring for their own relatives, but lacked the knowledge to do this effectively. Much attention was given to 'putting the patient's room in nursing order', with reference to hygiene, ventilation and light. Nurses also educated people about the danger posed by flies and other pests. First aid and emergency interventions were also part of district nursing work. In the days before disposables, all equipment had to be sterilised in the home, either by boiling on a stove or heating in an oven. Used dressings were burned on the household fire (Figures 1.3 and 1.4).

The first nurses' homes were rented flats or cottages, but by the 1930s dedicated nurses' homes were being designed and built all over the country. These often included a 'district room' where a nurse could see patients, as well as stores for medical supplies and a garage (Figures 1.5 and 1.6). The earliest district nurses either walked to visit their patients or used a pony and trap. In the early twentieth century, bicycles were widely adopted, replaced in turn by motor scooters and small cars. In rural areas, where doctors were often remote, nurses were given additional responsibility. Many district nurses were trained as midwives and, after 1920, as health visitors too.

At least until the 1950s most district nurses were single women, living in nurses' homes provided by local nursing associations. The nursing associations also employed the nurses in the days before the NHS; salaries were funded by donations and subscriptions. Nurses often had to collect fees from their patients, something that many nurses found very uncomfortable. From 1948, district nurses were employed first by local authorities and then by community healthcare organisations that have continued to evolve as part of the NHS ever since.

Post-1948, in the early years of the NHS, much district nursing work involved combating infectious diseases such as tuberculosis, as well as caring for people with diabetes, cancer, bronchitis, or mental illness, and people who were disabled through accident or other cause. End-of-life care and wound care was very important, as was the coordination of other services. Modern district nursing has continued to evolve to meet the needs of people in their own homes, leading and coordinating the work of the multidisciplinary team. Today, as specialist practitioners, district nurses play a vital role to play in enabling people to live in greater comfort in their own homes, preventing unnecessary suffering and distress and promoting independence.

2 History of the Queen's Nursing Institute

Matthew Bradby

Figure 2.1 Insignia of Queen Victoria's Jubilee Institute for Nurses, 1887. Source: Queen's Nursing Institute.

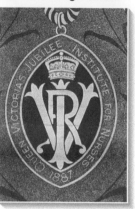

Figure 2.2 Queen's Nurse's Outdoor Uniform, 1905. Source: Queen's Nursing Institute.

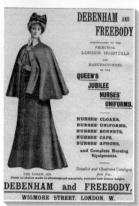

Figure 2.3 Uniform hat for Queen's Nurses, 1913. Source: Queen's Nursing Institute.

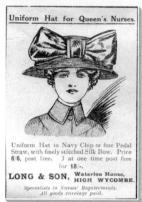

Figure 2.4 Queen's Nursing Institute badge for Jamaican nurses. Source: Queen's Nursing Institute.

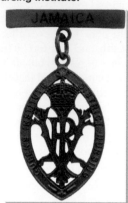

Figure 2.5 Queen's Nurse's indoor uniform, 1943. Source: Queen's Nursing Institute.

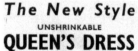
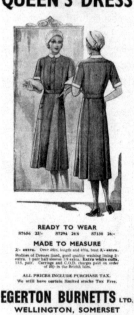

Figure 2.6 Queen's Institute of District Nursing logo, 1928. Source: Queen's Nursing Institute.

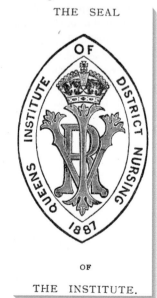

Figure 2.7 Queen's Nursing Institute logo, 1973. Source: Queen's Nursing Institute.

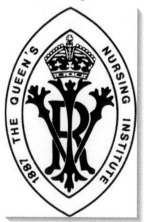

Figure 2.8 Modern Queen's Nurse badge. Source: Queen's Nursing Institute.

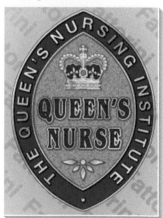

District Nursing at a Glance, First Edition. Edited by Matthew Bradby.
© 2022 John Wiley & Sons Ltd. Published 2022 by John Wiley & Sons Ltd.

The Queen's Nursing Institute is a registered charity, created to organise the training of district nurses in the UK. It traces its origins to 1887 with a grant of £70,000 by Queen Victoria and a Royal Charter in 1889 named it Queen Victoria's Jubilee Institute for Nurses. Its original objectives were the 'training, support, maintenance of women to act as nurses for the sick poor and the establishment . . . of a home or homes for nurses and generally the promotion and provision of improved means of nursing the sick poor.' William Rathbone, who had pioneered the concept of district nursing in 1859, and Florence Nightingale were closely involved in the creation of the new charity. Queen Victoria was the charity's first Patron in a tradition that has continued to the present day: Her Majesty Queen Elizabeth II became Patron in 2002.

District nurses who undertook the Institute's training and passed its examination were called Queen's Nurses and were entitled to wear the badge and insignia of the Institute (Figures 2.1–2.3). Early training contained a broad range of subjects, including sanitary reform, health education, ventilation, water supply, diet, infectious diseases, sexual health, and the feeding and care of newborn infants (in this period, infant mortality was around 154 per 1000 live births). Queen's Nurses began visiting schools in London when it was realised that school children suffered from a wide variety of ailments made worse by lack of treatment – a key milestone in the development of modern school nursing.

The Institute's Council – its governing body – laid down the 'Conditions of Affiliation' for district nursing associations, the local charities that employed nurses until 1948. These conditions included the qualifications required of Queen's Nurses, including training at an approved hospital or infirmary for at least a year; approved training in district nursing for at least six months; training in nursing of mothers and infants after childbirth (subsequently, this contributed to the development of the health visitor profession). Nurses in country districts also had to have three months' training in midwifery. Nursing was carried out under the direction of medical practitioners, and services were confined to the poor, 'while not excluding cases of such patients as are able to make some small contribution.' Nurses were 'strictly forbidden to interfere in any way with the religious opinions of patients or members of their families'.

The idea of district nursing spread rapidly in areas of British colonialism and other regions overseas. The Victorian Order of Nurses for Canada was founded in 1897, while in Australia the 'Bush' Nursing Association was founded in 1911. In the United States, the Boston district nursing association was founded in 1886 and the National Organisation for Public Health Nursing by 1912.

The King Edward VII Order of Nurses was founded in South Africa in 1913. European countries also experimented with the district nursing model. In many cases, trained district nurses from Britain and Ireland helped to staff these overseas organisations. In 1909 the Jubilee Congress of District Nursing was held in Liverpool, attended by delegates from all over the world. District nursing had become an international movement.

After the Second World War, the Institute helped arrange for 50 Greek women to come to Britain for nurse training. In 1955, 41 Queen's Nurses were appointed to posts abroad. The January 1958 Queen's Nurses' magazine listed overseas district nursing services that had started in Malta (1946), Jamaica (1957) (Figure 2.4), Singapore (1956), Nigeria (1954), Tanganyika (1957) and Kenya (1956) in collaboration with authorities in those countries. Nurses from those countries came to the Institute for training, some returning home and others staying in the UK. Delegations came from France, Brazil, Turkey, India, Greece and Finland to find out more about the administration and training of district nurses in Britain.

In 1948 the NHS began operating and the employment of district nurses fell to local authorities. Local district nursing organisations no longer had a purpose and quickly ceased to exist; however over 50 accredited training centres training 700 nurses a year were still affiliated to the Institute (Figure 2.5). The Institute finally ceased to offer full training for district nurses in 1968 when the qualification was absorbed into higher education, and the title of Queen's Nurse lapsed.

The charity was renamed the Queen's Institute of District Nursing in 1928 (Figure 2.6) and the Queen's Nursing Institute (QNI) in 1973 (Figure 2.7). Today the QNI operates in England, Wales and Northern Ireland. The Queen's Nursing Institute Scotland (QNIS) is a separate charity with its headquarters in Edinburgh. The Queen's Institute of District Nursing in Ireland is an affiliated charity in the Republic of Ireland.

The title of Queen's Nurse (QN) was reintroduced in 2007 as a means of reinforcing the professional identity of community nurses. Today the QN title is no longer restricted to district nurses: any nurse who has worked in the community for 5 years is eligible to apply (Figure 2.8). The Institute also offers educational bursaries, awards, professional development and financial assistance to nurses in need. The charity also works to influence healthcare policy, supports innovation and practice development, undertakes research, publishes reports on community nursing practice and holds regular educational events, including an annual conference and general meeting for all Queen's Nurses.

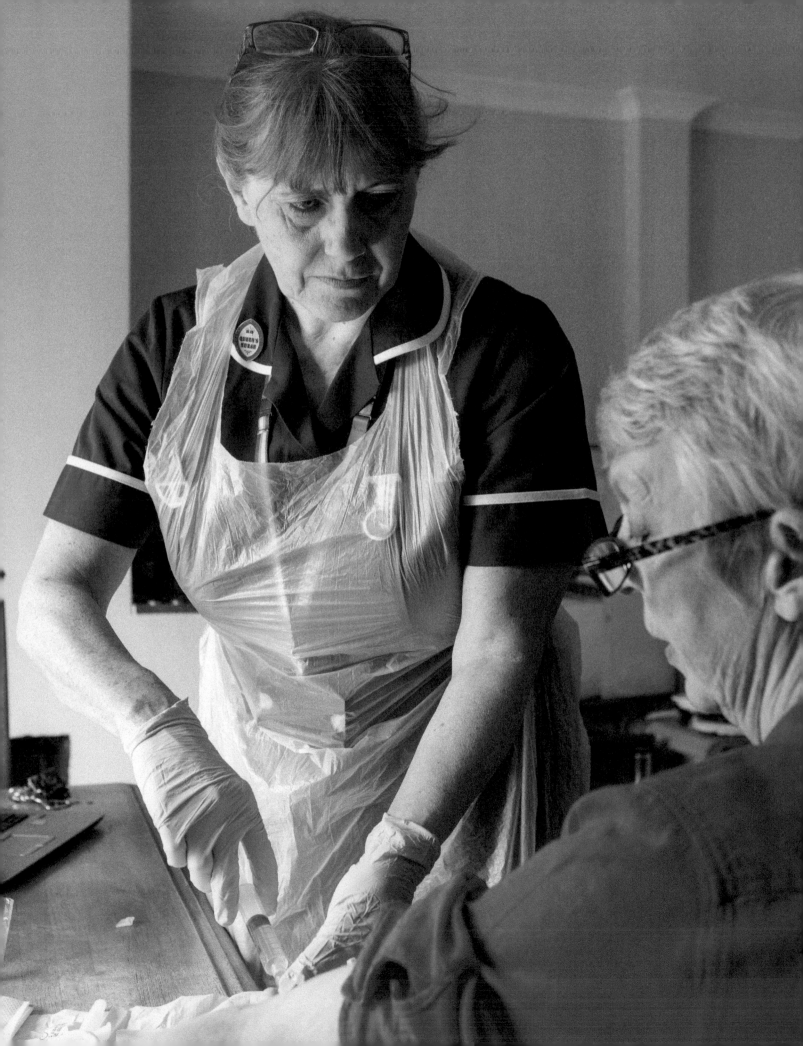

The learning environment

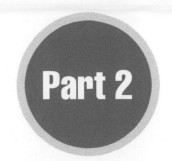

Part 2

Chapters

3 Preparation for a learning environment in the community

Shirley Willis, QN

Figure 3.1 The three pillars supporting learning within the community setting.

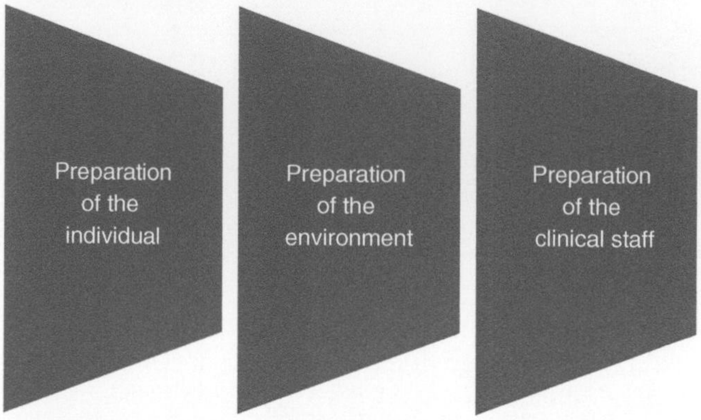

Preparation of the individual

Preparation of the environment

Preparation of the clinical staff

Figure 3.2 Individual learning styles.

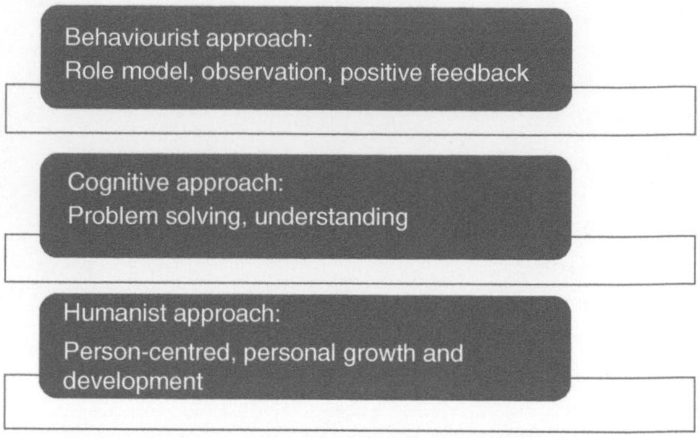

Behaviourist approach:
Role model, observation, positive feedback

Cognitive approach:
Problem solving, understanding

Humanist approach:
Person-centred, personal growth and development

Figure 3.3 Quality in community education.

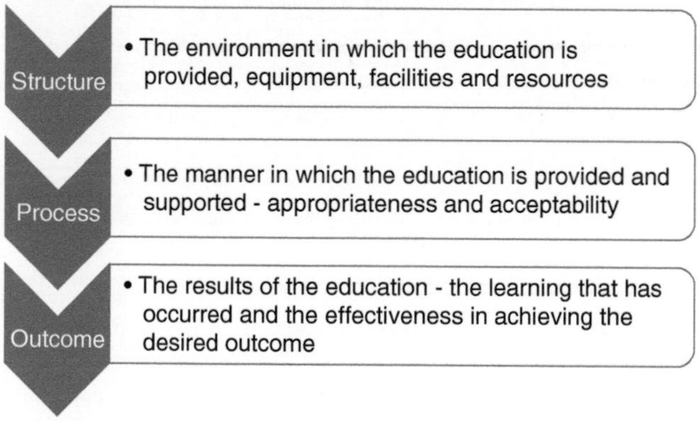

Structure
• The environment in which the education is provided, equipment, facilities and resources

Process
• The manner in which the education is provided and supported - appropriateness and acceptability

Outcome
• The results of the education - the learning that has occurred and the effectiveness in achieving the desired outcome

Table 3.1 Elements contributing to effective clinical supervisor–student relationships.

Clinical placement supervisor	Student
• Identify expectations	• Realistic expectations
• Professional approach	• Professional approach
• Set boundaries	• Willingness and commitment
• Dedicated time for the student	• Reflective learner
• Competence and experience	• Self-awareness
• Credible role model	• Understands own learning needs
• Questioning	• Questioning
• Facilitates learning	

District Nursing at a Glance, First Edition. Edited by Matthew Bradby.
© 2022 John Wiley & Sons Ltd. Published 2022 by John Wiley & Sons Ltd.

Caring for patients within their home environment, which could be a private house or a residential or nursing home setting, provides the nursing student with a number of unique learning opportunities. In preparing to learn within this very diverse and often challenging setting, it may be helpful to begin by considering the learning opportunities in terms of the skills that the student may be able to develop:

- *Communication skills*: Talking to patients, family members, carers and other health professionals in an environment where the nurse is the 'visitor'.
- *Observational skills*: Recognising the challenges that the patient may face in achieving concordance with any identified plan of care.
- *Consultation skills*: History taking and information gathering in order to inform the development of a care plan. It is important to consider the limitations of the environment and the absence of many of the structures and support services that may be taken for granted within the acute healthcare setting in order to inform the plan.
- *Presentation skills*: Presenting information both formally and informally in a manner that can be understood by the particular audience and is appropriate to the setting.
- *Flexibility, adaptability and competency skills*: Being able to carry out skills competently and effectively whilst adapting to the challenges of the environment.
- *Evaluation skills*: Considering outcomes of care in terms of the patient themselves, the delivery of the service in this setting, and in relation to the organisation's objectives and targets.

Although these skills are all transferable to other healthcare settings, learning within the community setting allows the practitioner to really develop these 'generalist' skills towards a more 'specialist' level, with clear benefits to patient care.

In order to be able to take full advantage of these learning opportunities, preparing to learn within this generalist/specialist arena will pay dividends in terms of both personal and professional development. Preparation for practice could be considered from a number of different perspectives relating to the individual student, the environment of care, and the clinical staff working in the practice area (Figure 3.1).

Individual learning

For the individual student, preparing to learn within the community setting may be guided by asking a number of questions:

- What are my personal learning and development needs at this point in time?
- What is my own learning style (Figure 3.2)?
- What do I understand by the term 'community'?
- What are my expectations of the community setting as an environment for learning?

- What knowledge/skills/experience can I bring to the community setting to enhance and maximise my learning experience?

In answering these questions it may be helpful to use a structured framework, such as the Strengths/Weaknesses/Opportunities/Concerns approach, to guide your decision-making.

The environment of care

It could be argued that any care environment that is clinically effective will also be an effective learning environment. However, a conscious effort is required in order to ensure that a clinical setting provides both students and practitioners with a safe and worthwhile learning experience. In ensuring quality within the learning environment it is helpful to consider the structure, process, and outcome of the learning experience (Figure 3.3).

In accordance with the Standards for pre-registration nursing programmes (Nursing and Midwifery Council, 2018a), it is a responsibility of the educational provider to ensure that students are provided with the opportunity to experience a wide variety of clinical experiences. Working together with clinical practice partners, students will be able to develop to meet the required standards of performance expected of a qualified nurse. Robust working relationships between educational and clinical staff are fundamental to ensuring that the learning environment is maintained.

Clinical simulation also plays a part in supporting preparation for clinical learning, giving students the opportunity to practise skills and 'make mistakes' in a safe environment, which would not be acceptable within clinical practice. Participating in community clinical simulation learning prior to going out into clinical practice allows the learner to be more aware of the role of decision-making and problem-solving skills, through reflection and debriefing, and to recognise environmental cues which will support the learner to contribute to holistic assessment in practice.

Clinical staff

This final element in the learning triad has a crucial role to play in ensuring a positive learning experience for students and practitioners. Acting as a supervisor and role model is fundamental to nursing practice and is recognised as a role for which there is a formal preparation process. Learners in the community setting need to be supported by an identified member of the clinical team and their goal is to empower students to have the confidence to take responsibility for their own learning.

Establishing a trusting working relationship between the student and clinical placement supervisor is fundamental to achieving a meaningful learning experience (Table 3.1). The community setting provides excellent opportunities for the development of interpersonal relationships as work is very much one-to-one, both with patients as well as when working closely with mentors in the home setting.

4 Providing student placements in the community

Irene Cooke, QN and Deborah Haydock, QN

Figure 4.1   Examples of alternative practice placements.

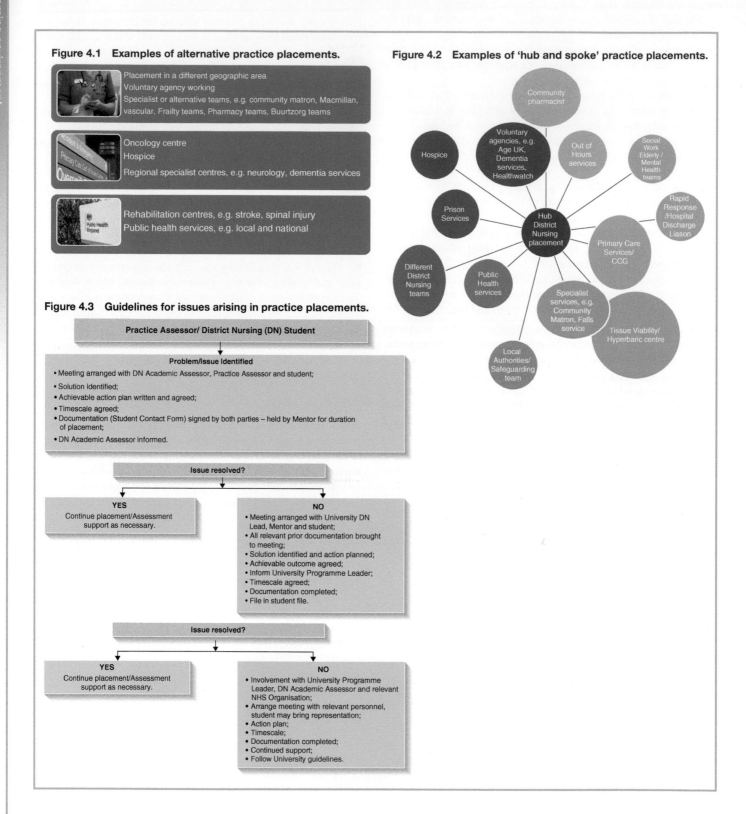

Placement in a different geographic area
Voluntary agency working
Specialist or alternative teams, e.g. community matron, Macmillan, vascular, Frailty teams, Pharmacy teams, Buurtzorg teams

Oncology centre
Hospice
Regional specialist centres, e.g. neurology, dementia services

Rehabilitation centres, e.g. stroke, spinal injury
Public health services, e.g. local and national

Figure 4.2   Examples of 'hub and spoke' practice placements.

- Community pharmacist
- Voluntary agencies, e.g. Age UK, Dementia services, Healthwatch
- Out of Hours services
- Social Work Elderly / Mental Health teams
- Hospice
- Prison Services
- Hub District Nursing placement
- Rapid Response /Hospital Discharge Liason
- Primary Care Services/ CCG
- Different District Nursing teams
- Public Health services
- Specialist services, e.g. Community Matron, Falls service
- Tissue Viability/ Hyperbaric centre
- Local Authorities/ Safeguarding team

Figure 4.3   Guidelines for issues arising in practice placements.

Practice Assessor/ District Nursing (DN) Student

↓

Problem/Issue Identified
- Meeting arranged with DN Academic Assessor, Practice Assessor and student;
- Solution identified;
- Achievable action plan written and agreed;
- Timescale agreed;
- Documentation (Student Contact Form) signed by both parties – held by Mentor for duration of placement;
- DN Academic Assessor informed.

↓

Issue resolved?

YES
Continue placement/Assessment support as necessary.

NO
- Meeting arranged with University DN Lead, Mentor and student;
- All relevant prior documentation brought to meeting;
- Solution identified and action planned;
- Achievable outcome agreed;
- Inform University Programme Leader;
- Timescale agreed;
- Documentation completed;
- File in student file.

↓

Issue resolved?

YES
Continue placement/Assessment support as necessary.

NO
- Involvement with University Programme Leader, DN Academic Assessor and relevant NHS Organisation;
- Arrange meeting with relevant personnel, student may bring representation;
- Action plan;
- Timescale;
- Documentation completed;
- Continued support;
- Follow University guidelines.

District Nursing at a Glance, First Edition. Edited by Matthew Bradby.
© 2022 John Wiley & Sons Ltd. Published 2022 by John Wiley & Sons Ltd.

District nursing students undertaking the specialist practice community programme must demonstrate higher levels of judgement, discretion and decision-making in clinical care. There are four key domains of specialist practice:

• Clinical practice
• Care and programme management
• Clinical practice development
• Clinical practice leadership.

The educational curriculum for the district nursing programme must be based upon these four key domains, which must be achieved within theoretical modules and practice over a minimum of 32 weeks. The purpose of the practice placement is to ensure that students are exposed to Nursing and Midwifery Council (NMC) core and specialist competencies through individualised bespoke placements, which enables students to safely practise and achieve competency and autonomy in their professional programme. The NMC (Nursing and Midwifery Council, 2018b) set out the expectations for the learning, support and supervision of students in the practice environment, including how students are assessed for theory and practice. All students on an NMC-approved programme, including district nursing students, must be supervised in practice by an NMC-registered nurse who understands the proficiencies and programme outcomes they are supporting students to achieve. In addition, all students on NMC-approved post-registration programmes are assigned to a nominated practice assessor in accordance with relevant programme standards. The higher education institution (HEI) is also responsible for allocating a nominated academic assessor who works in partnership with the practice assessor to evaluate and recommend the student for progression, in line with programme standards.

Students must document their learning within practice using a practice portfolio, as this is the vehicle for practice assessment for the duration of the programme. The practice portfolio should be developed throughout the duration of the programme. The portfolio should be used to guide and structure the students learning in practice, providing the opportunity for the student to work closely with their practice assessor and practice supervisor in order to identify learning opportunities that will meet agreed NMC competencies.

Regular meetings between the student, academic assessor and practice assessor/practice supervisor are essential for successful practice portfolio development. Meetings should occur at specified times within the programme, such as an initial meeting, mid-point and a summative meeting. The portfolio is as important as theoretical assignments as it provides evidence that supports the assessment of practice. Evidence must be provided for each of the four practice assessment domains, and all competencies must be successfully met. The practice portfolio should act as a medium for critical discourse between student, practice supervisor, practice assessor and academic assessor.

Placements should provide exposure to a range of learning opportunities. This may be achieved through the use of the 'hub and spoke' model, which can be adapted to local need, whilst building upon students' prior knowledge, skills and experience. An alternative practice placement of a minimum of one week is suggested as good practice to enable the student to experience geographic differences in service delivery and a range of specialist services (Figure 4.1).

Both strategies enhance the students' knowledge and skills and their understanding of inter-professional and multi-agency working. The district nursing team where the student is placed is the 'Hub' and this is the focus for the majority of the learning: the student would be exposed to the key domains of clinical practice, care and programme management, clinical practice development and clinical practice leadership. The 'Spoke' provides eclectic and individualised learning opportunities. Finding new ways in which to engage with the voluntary sector, support patient choice and sharing leadership with patients will be an increasing focus as district nurses find themselves involved in new care delivery models. Spoke placements with charitable organisations may prove significant in understanding how communities empower groups (Figure 4.2).

User centrality is pivotal in the NHS strategy, and involvement of service users in healthcare improves partnerships, access to services and better service planning. Practice assessors and practice supervisors should identify patients or client groups with whom the student has contact, and ask them to complete user feedback on the student's performance. Service user feedback should be sought at least once during each semester. This should act as a catalyst for discussion between the student, practice supervisor and practice assessor.

It is strongly advised that a placement contract is formulated between the student and the practice supervisor and practice assessor, as this may prevent problems arising in practice and can assist in the development of learning opportunities. Contracting ensures a structured approach to meeting the programme learning outcomes, allowing for negotiation and the development of a student-centred placement experience that fosters professional development. The contract also facilitates realistic planning and the setting of achievable goals. Regular review of the contract allows for formative assessments and action plans to be revisited and changed as required. Occasionally there may be issues in practice and these need to be monitored and concerns actioned (Figure 4.3).

During specialist practice, it is recommended that a series of action learning sets are undertaken. These action learning sets can be inter-professional, facilitating understanding of professional roles and responsibilities, which may help to support the delivery of an integrated care workforce (Gilburt, 2016). The process is based on the idea that effective learning and development has to be about real problems in real life with real people (Raelin, 1998). Through action learning, individuals learn with and from each other by working on real problems and reflecting on their own experiences (Haydock and Evers, 2014).

The benefits of action learning are:

• Greater breadth in understanding collaboration and inter-professional learning to build up relationships in community nursing practice.
• Increased ability to analyse ambiguous situations and solve complex problems.
• Enhanced capacity to understand and initiate changes that increases the focus on what makes a difference in a situation.
• Better ability to be more action focused and proactive in delivering results.
• Enhanced self-awareness and appreciation of personal impact on others, contributing to improved ability to work with others.
• Developed flexibility in responding to changing situations
• Shared knowledge and learning.

Students are able to listen to and reflect upon others' experiences, ask questions, gaining different perspectives (Pedler and Abbott, 2008). When members share information and resources, it provides practical and emotional support. The student and the practice assessor and practice supervisor should actively work together to participate in the action learning sets, which may be recorded and included as evidence in the portfolio.

Supporting nursing students in the community

Josephine Gray, QN

Box 5.1 Examples of clinical skill experiences students may undertake during their community placement.

- Care of the diabetic patient, blood glucose monitoring and insulin administration.
- Continence advice and assessment and knowledge of incontinence products, order and supply.
- Tissue viability. Methods of wound assessment and correct choice of dressings. Venous and arterial leg ulcer management. Doppler assessment and compression bandaging. Pressure damage prevention and treatment and ordering of pressure-relieving equipment.
- Medicines management and community prescriptions. Administration of intramuscular and subcutaneous injections. Application of creams and lotions, eye and ear drops. PV and PR medications administration and use.
- End-of-life care at home and in residential home. Syringe driver management. Care at time of death, verification of death and support for family and friends.
- Intravenous medication administration. Care of central lines and cannula. Chemotherapy disconnection.
- Care of patients living with dementia in their own home and in residential care.
- Lone working, autonomous practice and insight into safety awareness in the community.
- Teaching professional carers specific tasks under a shared care protocol.

Box 5.2 Members of the multidisciplinary team that students may meet or work with during their community placement.

- General practitioners
- Practice nurses
- Community physiotherapists
- Community occupational therapists
- Community psychiatric nurses
- Podiatrists
- Practice managers
- Community matrons
- Specialist nurses (e.g. respiratory, cardiac rehabilitation, heart failure, Parkinsons)
- Community hospice nurses
- Health visitors
- School nurses
- Community midwives

District Nursing at a Glance, First Edition. Edited by Matthew Bradby.
© 2022 John Wiley & Sons Ltd. Published 2022 by John Wiley & Sons Ltd.

In recent years there has been a shift from care in hospital to more care being provided in the community, a move emphasised in the *NHS Long Term Plan*. In view of this, schools of nursing have had to adapt their teaching programmes so that students are prepared for this transition. Within the last few years, community placements have changed so that students can experience community nursing in all 3 years of their training.

Each learning establishment will have a different programme based on the fundamentals set down by the Nursing and Midwifery Council and each placement will differ in experience as community nursing is so diverse; however, the basic principles remain.

Year 1 placement

Year 1 focuses on the fundamental basics of nursing, all of which should be achievable in the community (Box 5.1). For some students, it will be their very first placement so they will need extra support. Up to 50% of this placement will be spent with their workplace mentor and the remaining time will be with other team members and working with other professionals in the multidisciplinary team (Box 5.2). They will be introduced to the everyday working of a community nursing team and experience the basics of community care. The mentor will introduce some of the key aspects of nursing during this placement.

The first action when working with the student will be to set out learning objectives. These will be a combination of both the fundamentals of nursing below and clinical tasks and skills.

Fundamentals of nursing

- *Reflection*: Students will be expected to complete many reflective pieces during their training. This will be introduced from the beginning of their course and they will be expected to complete at least one reflection during each community placement.
- *Portfolio*: All nurses in training will be expected to complete a portfolio. Evidence from community placement must be collected, referenced and included in this.
- *Multidisciplinary working*: There are opportunities to work with multidisciplinary teams working in the community. The student will learn how shared care is provided in order to maximise a high standard of patient care.
- *Record keeping*: Meeting patients who have numerous sets of notes can be confusing. Most electronic NHS records should soon be within the same set of case notes. However, care agencies will always keep separate documentation.

Experience the patient-centred care approach

The student will practice assessments, complete medicine charts and care plans under supervision, and identify how this information is shared with other disciplines.

Challenging situations

The student may encounter difficult family dynamics, which can be heightened in times of illness and at the end of life, and will also visit home environments that are between the two extremes of poverty and wealth. The student must learn to be tolerant and non-judgemental. The student will experience the dynamic of being a guest in someone's home. They will also understand the role of a family carer and the importance they have on a patient's wellbeing and ability to remain at home. Students will practise how to raise a vulnerable adult alert with social services. Students must be made aware of the lone working policy.

Communication

Effective communication, verbal and non-verbal, will be explained and used. The student will learn effective responses to telephone enquiries, triage and information sharing, and maintain confidentiality especially in families when a patient does not want to share information with loved ones or in a shared office. They will experience many issues regarding language barriers and learn strategies to manage this. They will be involved in constructive feedback to other agencies involved.

Incident management

The student will experience the need for infection prevention in patients' homes that may not be hygienically clean. They will need to learn to identify potential risks and discuss them with families, and may need to work in areas that have manual handling problems such as low beds, cramped environments, and poor lighting. The student will learn to recognise problems that could arise if it was necessary to perform resuscitation in the community without complex equipment and often in confined places.

Health promotion

The student will learn to give advice about diet, nutrition and hydration, discuss weight management and healthy eating. They will learn about tools used to monitor wellbeing, clinical waste collection and pressure damage prevention.

Year 2

When students undertake a second year placement, the emphasis is to enhance and reaffirm all the knowledge they have gained from their first year placement and identify areas of care that may not have been undertaken in that placement. It will introduce them to more complex skills.

Year 3

In the third year, students will undertake a management placement and will be assigned a small caseload of their own. This gives them the opportunity to consolidate what they have previously learnt and to lead patient care as a named nurse. They will develop their triage skills and learn how to be a coordinator, leading allocation of patients and handover. They will be given more complex care roles and more in-depth assessments. It will establish them as autonomous practitioners and part of a team. It will support them into being effective leaders, learning the aspects of good leadership and how to positively respond to change. They will be expected to have an in-depth knowledge around drivers for change and government directives for care in the community.

Mentorship and preceptorship

Meriel Chudleigh, QN

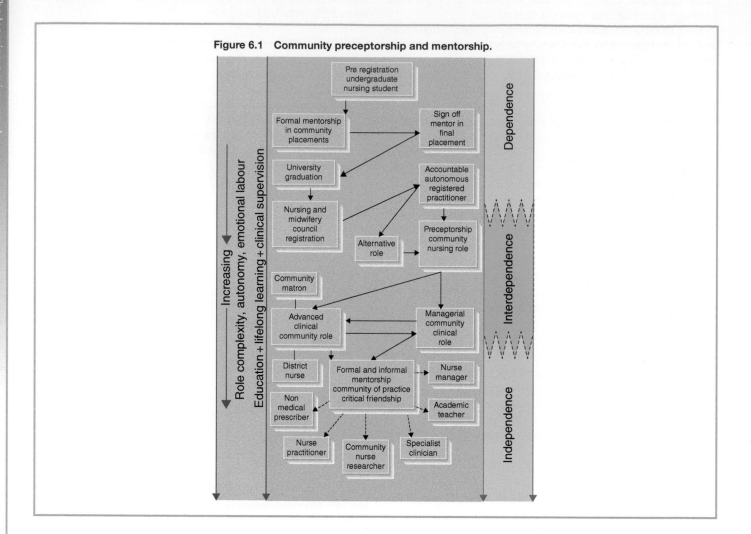

Figure 6.1 Community preceptorship and mentorship.

District Nursing at a Glance, First Edition. Edited by Matthew Bradby.
© 2022 John Wiley & Sons Ltd. Published 2022 by John Wiley & Sons Ltd.

Nursing is changing and the expectations of service users, healthcare professionals and society are rising. The demographic need and demand for 'care closer to home' is driving a move to minimise hospital contact and optimise community health support. Undergraduate nursing students spend significant amounts of mentor-supported practice time in community settings to prepare them for these challenging and rewarding roles. From the point of registration, all healthcare professionals are autonomous, accountable practitioners, but the first weeks and months in a community role are aided by the support of experienced colleagues, either informally or through preceptor or mentor facilitation (Figure 6.1).

Preceptorship

A preceptee is a registered healthcare practitioner entering a new community role, supported by the formal process of preceptorship. A preceptee could be a newly qualified registrant, a professional returning to registration following a break in practice, a nurse entering a new part of the Nursing and Midwifery Council (NMC) register, or an overseas nurse starting a role in the UK.

A preceptor is a formally responsible nurse (on the same part of the NMC register) supporting a preceptee through role modelling, facilitating of learning and guidance throughout the community preceptorship. Effective preceptors are experienced peers with leadership and communication skills and a desire to support professional development.

A preceptorship involves a formal transition period of supported learning and may involve some supernumerary time. It may last from two weeks to four months or more, depending on the situation and needs of the preceptee. The aim of the preceptorship is to develop the competence and confident of the preceptee. An initial set of objectives provides a planning focus and frequent contact between preceptee and preceptor occurs, particularly during the first weeks. Contacts may involve discussion to optimise action plans, reflection on practice and receiving feedback on progress. The preceptorship may involve additional skills training: time shadowing a role model, observation of practice, clinical supervision and activities to integrate the preceptee into the primary care multidisciplinary team. Structured learning opportunities in groups or online alongside one-to-one contact with the preceptor enables optimal progress and effective use of resources.

The preceptor also benefits from the experience in facilitating community staff development, progress in lifelong learning and evidence to aid career progression. Both preceptor and preceptee gain from the relationship; however, it requires the development of trust, reflective skills and honesty to use the opportunity to its full potential.

Employing organisations are responsible for implementing and supporting preceptorship frameworks, including learning objectives and competencies appropriate to the role. Preceptorship is considered to be separate from organisation induction processes and mandatory certification. Employers benefit from preceptorships too, through increased staff satisfaction, role competence and confidence, and improved community staff retention.

Mentorship

Mentorship is a two-way relationship intended to support, develop and assess learning in practice and individual personal and professional development.

A mentor is an expert or experienced practitioner who is either selected by the mentee or allocated to the mentor role of facilitator and in some circumstances as assessor. A mentee is a person requiring support and supervision to aid personal and professional development. The NMC requires an allocated registered mentor to support and assess undergraduate students during each practice placement. During the final pre-registration placement a skilled and responsible 'sign off' mentor assesses competence and confirms that the applicant is professionally ready to join the register.

Other less formal mentorship roles are also present in UK community healthcare and these offer both the 'mentee' and the 'mentor' development opportunities. Mentorship may be required to fulfil certain course or role requirements, or help develop leadership, management, advanced practice, research or teaching abilities. Learning in practice involves internal personal change and the mentor initially provides support and guidance, leading gradually to increasing role competence and confidence. A dynamic relationship develops between mentor and mentee arising from regular contact and focussed discussion of needs, concerns and interests.

Initially, a mentee will be in a dependent position but this should develop (particularly in post-registration situations) to a more equal professional relationship with mutual beneficial growth. A critical friendship can develop the relationship further to enhance the opportunity to challenge practices and values, stimulate healthy discussion and drive innovative progress.

In community settings, mentorship has particular relevance due to the potential challenges of working alone in patient's own homes or in roles where more autonomy is required. Dealing with uncertainty and making safe independent clinical management decisions involves understanding the complex interaction of physical, social and psychological aspects of care. This exposure to new learning experiences drives emotional and professional development. The interpersonal skills of the mentor are important to the success of the relationship and the optimal use of the opportunity. Ultimately both the mentor and mentee come through a process of change and are better equipped to understand the challenges and opportunities of community healthcare.

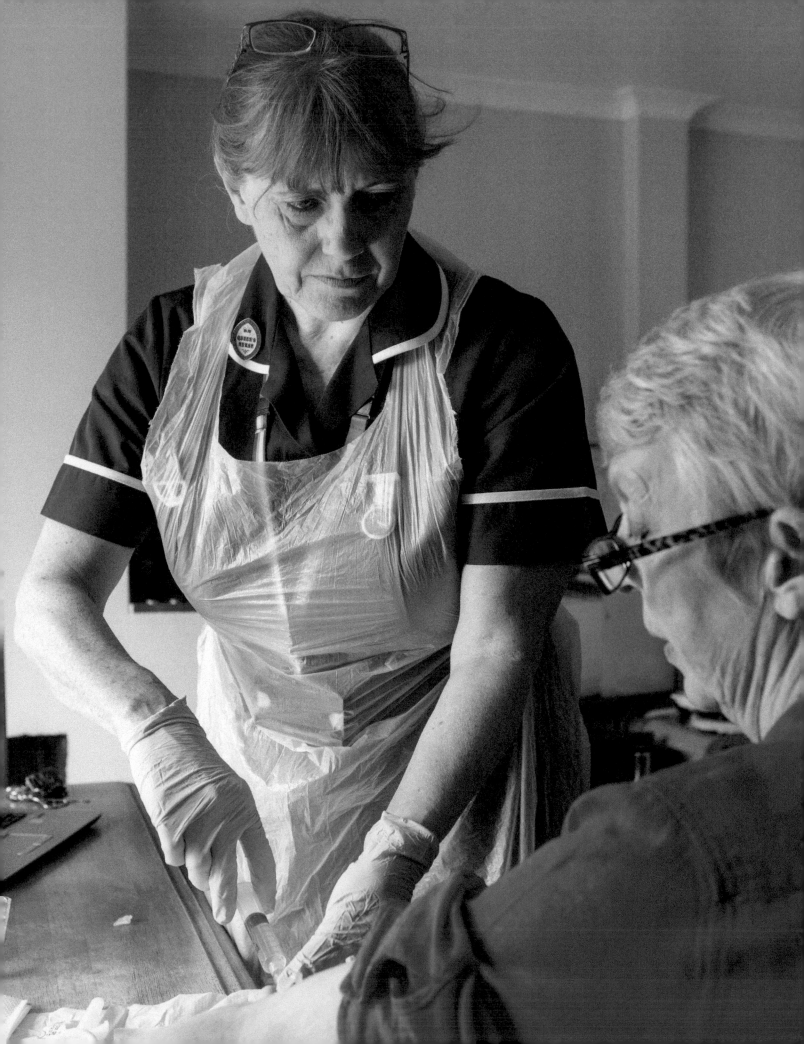

Working in the community

Part 3

Chapters

7 The role of the district nurse: autonomous practice

Matthew Peasey, QN

Figure 7.1 A district nurse carrying equipment from a patient's home.

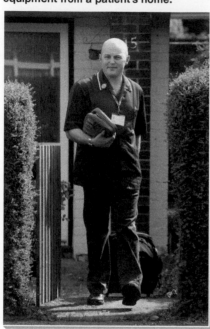

Figure 7.2 A district nurse on her rounds.

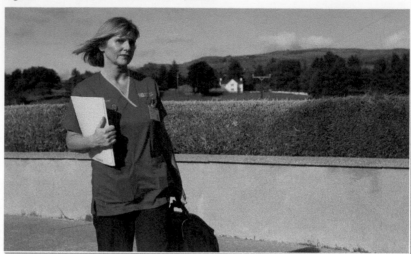

Figure 7.3 The novice to expert continuum.

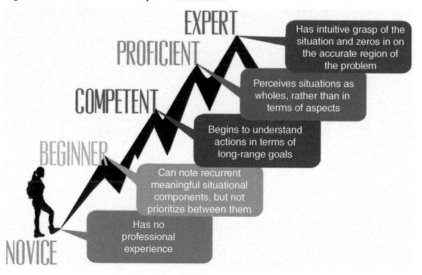

EXPERT — Has intuitive grasp of the situation and zeros in on the accurate region of the problem

PROFICIENT — Perceives situations as wholes, rather than in terms of aspects

COMPETENT — Begins to understand actions in terms of long-range goals

BEGINNER — Can note recurrent meaningful situational components, but not prioritize between them

NOVICE — Has no professional experience

District Nursing at a Glance, First Edition. Edited by Matthew Bradby.
© 2022 John Wiley & Sons Ltd. Published 2022 by John Wiley & Sons Ltd.

The title 'district nurse' is widely and often incorrectly used by nursing colleagues, even by nurses working within community/district nursing services themselves. In turn this has meant that patient understanding and respect of the district nurse role and level of responsibility has been eroded. However, district nurses and their community nursing colleagues remain an integral part of the community healthcare system, bringing healthcare closer to home and preventing unnecessary hospital admissions. The NHS England Long Term Plan (https://www.longtermplan.nhs.uk/) has reinforced how important district nurses will be to delivering healthcare closer to and within people's homes and communities (Figure 7.1).

Novice to expert

Traditionally, district nursing was an essential but somewhat isolated role in villages, towns and cities. These nurses unassumingly and diligently visited patients in their own homes, caring for families they often knew very well. They sought to maintain patients' ability to stay at home or to rehabilitate them, in the hope that nursing care would eventually no longer be needed. They achieved this by minimising the risk of harm, using their intuition and learned skills from experience with previous patients to constantly move care forward. Essentially, they became the leaders in supportive care and self-management (Figure 7.2).

Today, experienced district nurses who have undertaken the combined theory and practice programme run by universities in the UK will have developed and built on their existing knowledge and skills to become safe, autonomous and competent specialist practitioners. They initiate, lead and deliver contemporary district nursing practice with the assistance of a team that includes healthcare assistants and other practitioners.

Autonomous practice

The thought of a nurse becoming autonomous may be a challenging concept for some clinicians to get to grips with. However, you could argue that the concept of autonomous practice is basically a re-invention of the novice-to-expert continuum (Figure 7.3): district nurses have always assumed an autonomous role without acknowledging it. They have always worked independently of their medical colleagues, only asking for guidance once their own skill set is exhausted. They have been creative in finding solutions for patients' and carers' challenges and inspired them to move away from being largely dependent on the nurse, through a stage of being partially dependent until ultimately becoming independent. This is essentially autonomous practice, in that the nurse is steering care and taking responsibility for his or her own actions without constantly needing reassurance or guidance. These nurses have become expert decision-makers and are confident in their own abilities and conduct.

District nurses have blurred the lines of what was traditionally thought of as nursing practice. While maintaining their nursing mind-set, they have developed and moved closer to the practice of their medical colleagues. In today's practice, a district nurse is expected to have a broad perspective, sound decision-making ability and a strong foundation in nursing practice, and to be an expert team leader. They achieve this today in different ways to those of the past, but still they prove their ability and commitment to patient care.

Physical examination and prescribing

District nurses need to be skilled in undertaking physical examination and consultation structuring. By doing so they are able to gain the information they need to motivationally interview their patients and make sound decisions about their care. Increasingly, patients are looking to their district nurse for planned, personalised and holistic care of their health, knowing that they have the skills and knowledge to provide that care at home.

Nurses who complete the Nursing and Midwifery Council (NMC) Community Practitioner Nurse Prescribing course (v100 or v150) may prescribe from the Nurse Prescribers' Formulary for Community Practitioners. This includes appliances, dressings and some medicines. Those who have completed an Independent Nurse Prescribing Course (v200 or v300) are able to prescribe any medicine, provided it is within their competency. Those who have completed the supplementary part of the course are also able to prescribe against a clinical management plan. Hence, district nurses are assuming many of the roles that would traditionally have been within the GP's core domain. In the community, district nurses have been the guiding light in advancing autonomous practice and this trend has transferred into the hospital setting. Medical colleagues have come to trust the district nurse's decision-making ability and community teams are inspired to provide excellent, holistic patient care.

Summary

- Moving towards autonomous practice is a continuous process. By embracing the concept of life-long learning you become safe; do not be afraid to use your intuition.
- You must be able to develop confidence in working alone, as well as leading a team and be prepared to make tricky decisions.
- Seek further education in advanced physical examination skills and prescribing; consult with patients and negotiate on plans of care so they may make informed choices.
- Instigate evidence-based practice through motivational interviewing.
- Know your boundaries and limitations; do not be scared to ask for help or guidance as this will make you more credible and build your confidence.
- Inspire your colleagues, seek to influence the decision-making process and advocate for your patients' interests.
- Refer to Chapter 18 about lone working for more information about staying safe, acknowledging risk and team working.
- Working in the community may not be for you if you feel vulnerable working alone or dislike driving.
- Do not follow trends, policies and procedures blindly or deliver task-focused care.
- Remember your roots in nursing and do not be afraid to deliver basic nursing when required.
- Do not be afraid to challenge.

Evidence-based practice

Ben Bowers, QN

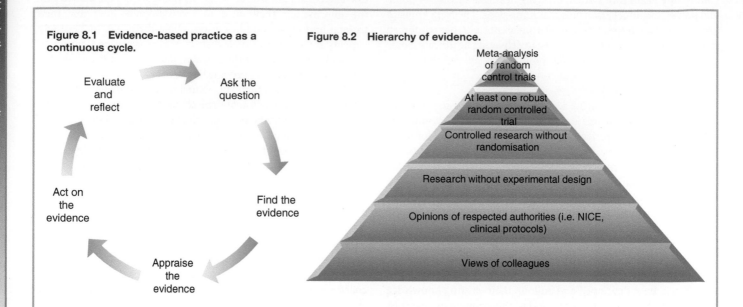

Figure 8.1   Evidence-based practice as a continuous cycle.

Ask the question → Find the evidence → Appraise the evidence → Act on the evidence → Evaluate and reflect → Ask the question

Figure 8.2   Hierarchy of evidence.

Meta-analysis of random control trials

At least one robust random controlled trial

Controlled research without randomisation

Research without experimental design

Opinions of respected authorities (i.e. NICE, clinical protocols)

Views of colleagues

Box 8.1   Useful evidence-based resources to access.

Systematic evidence review websites
- NICE clinical knowledge summaries http://cks.nice.org.uk/#?char=A
- Cochrane library http://www.cochranelibrary.com
- Bandolier http://www.bandolier.org.uk
- University of York Centre for Reviews and Dissemination http://www.crd.york.ac.uk/CRDWeb/

Journals and books
- Journals where papers are 'peer reviewed'
- Open access journals which are 'peer reviewed'
- Text books, e.g. *District Nursing Manual of Clinical Procedures*

Online database searches
- NICE evidence search http://www.evidence.nhs.uk
- OpenAthens account (giving free access to NHS staff to multiple health and nursing databases) http://www.openathens.net/nhs_users.php
- Google scholar (not as comprehensive as health/nursing-specific databases) https://scholar.google.co.uk
- Royal College of Nursing library resources (free access to a range of health and nursing databases for members) https://www.rcn.org.uk/development/library_and_heritage_services

Evidence-based guidance
- NICE http://www.nice.org.uk/Guidance
- Department of Health and Social Care https://www.gov.uk/government/publications
- Queen's Nursing Institute http://www.qni.org.uk/for_nurses/publications
- Royal College of Nursing http://www.rcn.org.uk/development/publications

Evidence-based mobile apps
- http://www.bestevidence.info/

Source: Bowers, B. (2018). Evidence-based practice in community nursing. *British Journal of Community Nursing* 23(7): 336–337.

There is an expectation that nurses use the most up-to-date and relevant evidence to inform decisions about their patients' care. Scientific and well-reasoned decisions improve patient care and make the best use of limited resources, and the application of evidence-based practice has always been a major driving force in district nursing. However, what is valued as evidence has changed to reflect societal and healthcare priorities. We currently prioritise empirical evidence demonstrating an intervention's clinical effectiveness (particularly its impact on patient outcomes); cost effectiveness; patient acceptability; safety, and acceptability to healthcare professionals (Figure 8.1). However, it is rare that the available evidence examines and demonstrates all these values.

Applying evidence in practice consists of five key consecutive steps:

1 Recognising there is a need for new information to answer a particular clinical question.
2 Searching and selecting a suitable range of evidence to answer the question.
3 Critically appraising this evidence.
4 Using the most applicable and best evidence, together with patient preferences, to inform clinical practice.
5 Evaluating the effectiveness of the intervention. This often leads to new clinical questions being formed and the process starts again.

Limitations in practice

Clinical decisions are not always based on the most up-to-date and valid available evidence. In a study of 82 primary care nurses, participants recalled using 67 different sources of information to inform their clinical decision-making (Thompson et al., 2005). However, participants were observed seeking information as a result of just 23% of their consultations. This almost always involved obtaining advice from colleagues.

A perception of lack of time to access information, and lack of knowledge in how to access it are key challenges in applying evidence-based practice (Thompson et al., 2005; Hanafin et al., 2014). For district nurses needing to make prompt clinical decisions with patients in the home, limited real-time access to evidence resources can be a substantial barrier to delivering evidence-based care. Phoning experienced peers or sourcing local policies and guidance is relatively quick. Conversely, these approaches narrow knowledge about what constitutes good evidence to certain perspectives and assumes that local policies and guidance are up-to-date.

Accessing resources

District nurses need answers to practical treatment decisions. Knowing where to access a robust range of evidence-based resources in community nursing is crucial. There is an array of useful resources including printed journals, books, online databases and evidence reviews (Box 8.1). In reality, the range and choice of evidence can be confusing in itself. Mobile phone apps offering easy-to-access and up-to-date evidence-based guidance are likely to play an increasingly important role in community practice.

For now, easily consumable and frequently updated online resources such as NICE Clinical Knowledge Summaries, NICE Pathways and Bandolier evidence reviews offer good starting points for gathering comprehensive evidence. The Cochrane database and University of York Centre for Reviews and Dissemination database provide systematic evidence-based reviews on key subjects. Well-written and informative peer-reviewed articles can prove a good way to identify key evidence on a subject.

The nature of under-identified community care clinical situations means it is often necessary to undertake literature searches (e.g. through CINAHL or BNI databases) and then critically review individual papers to inform evidence-based decision making. These can be accessed online through the likes of OpenAthens and Royal College of Nursing (RCN) membership library services. It is also feasible to use Google Scholar, though undertaking a search on this alone is not recommended, as it will give limited results and article access. Local NHS librarians are experts in undertaking literature searches (a specialist area in itself) and can provide invaluable help and guidance. NHS libraries often offer to help design and undertake literature searches, making the process much more efficient.

What constitutes good evidence?

Contemporary evidence-based reviews have an established hierarchy, valuing studies with objective reliability (Figure 8.2). Randomised controlled trials or evidence from large-scale clinical trials are prized well above descriptive studies, qualitative research or expert opinion. Yet in district nursing care, there is a scarcity of randomised controlled trial data for a multitude of reasons. These include the difficulties inherent in controlling variables in patients' own homes, limited research interest and funding, and the prevailing focus on studying the impact of interventions in hospital environments.

The evidence base is frequently drawn from a mixture of qualitative and small-scale quantitative studies, expert opinion and translating the results of hospital-based studies, each providing partial insights into what constitutes best practice. Using a multitude of different evidence sources has benefits for patient care because it does not overvalue the importance of randomised controlled trials (Mantzoukas, 2008). Although useful, evidence from randomised controlled trials does not lend itself readily to providing care in patients' homes where variable psychosocial factors play a crucial role. Well-designed qualitative studies can provide meaningful insights into patient preferences and complex processes of care.

Evidence-based practice must centre around patient preferences, desires and clinical judgements in individual situations (Jacobs et al., 2012). This is where communication and therapeutic relationship-building skills (the art of nursing) interplay profoundly with knowing what clinical intervention will be most effective (the science of nursing). In practice there are often several ways to undertake care, each with their advantages and limitations. Providing the patient is making an informed choice, and where care is evidence-based and regularly evaluated in partnership with the patient, care is likely to be clinically effective.

9 Communication

Claire Green, QN

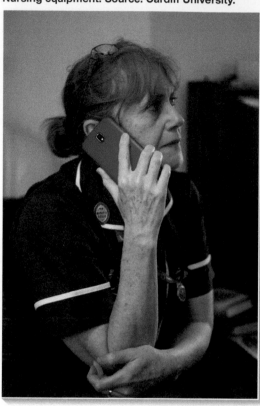

Figure 9.1   A mobile phone is a key piece of District Nursing equipment. Source: Cardiff University.

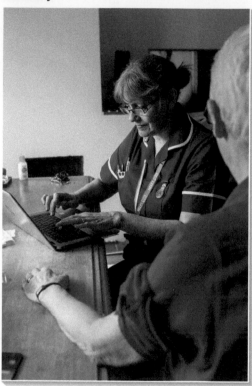

Figure 9.2   Working with a laptop or tablet to record and share patient notes. Source: Cardiff University.

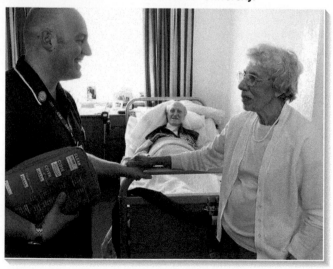

Figure 9.3   Developing good relationships with family members and carers is essential. Source: Cardiff University.

District Nursing at a Glance, First Edition. Edited by Matthew Bradby.
© 2022 John Wiley & Sons Ltd. Published 2022 by John Wiley & Sons Ltd.

ommunication, verbal or non-verbal, is at the heart of all our interactions in life. As nurses we are communicating daily between ourselves and other colleagues, with patients and their families and also with the wider community. Accurate communication is vital to ensure we give, receive and process information in a timely and appropriate way (Figure 9.1).

The first meeting with a patient can significantly influence any future relationship one has with them, so it is vitally important to introduce oneself at this time. A simple, 'Hello my name is . . .' or 'I'm . . .' is usually sufficient, but always be prepared to offer official identification and ensure they have your contact details. This initial meeting is also the time to find out what the patient prefers to be called; some are happy with first names from the start, whilst others may prefer to be addressed as 'Mr' or 'Mrs'. Always beware of using terms such as 'love' or 'dear'; these may be perfectly natural in one area but some patients may find being addressed like this condescending or patronising.

At the first visit to a patient, assess if they have any issues that could act as a barrier to effective communication. Are they hard of hearing, poorly sighted or blind, do they have a speech impediment? Is English their first language? Appropriate body language is also very important when entering someone else's home, and always be prepared to adapt your approach to the circumstances.

Simple things such as writing things down for patients who are hard of hearing may help; establish if they have a working hearing aid or if they need wax removing from their ear. For patients who are blind or poorly sighted there is a huge element of trust on their part to accept us for who we say we are and allow us into their homes. If their disability is known prior to a visit, then an initial telephone call may be useful as an introduction and to arrange a suitable time to visit. Patients who cannot speak may rely on talking devices or writing and it is important to give them time to express themselves (Figure 9.2).

Increasingly, district nurses are caring for people, often elderly, for whom English is not their first language. Family members are usually able to help translate but occasionally it may be necessary to enlist the help of an official interpreter. This may be necessary when trying to discuss complex care such as end-of-life care planning where technical terms may be used, or to ensure a discussion is relayed without bias or concealment, or because of gender issues.

Family and carers

The relationship with a relative or family member is of equal importance to that with the patient themselves. They can be an invaluable source of information about the patient, particularly if that person has dementia for example. Relatives can be concerned about what we will discuss with the patient, particularly if a recent cancer diagnosis has been given, where they may ask that this information is withheld. Whilst this may be appropriate initially, it is important not to collude with the family and withhold information, as it may have an impact on care delivery. Ensure that patients and their relatives understand any medical terminology that has been given to them; patients may have been told that they have a 'tumour' but not understand that this could indicate a cancer diagnosis (Figure 9.3).

It is important to reassure relatives that if a patient asks a direct question it will be answered as honestly and sensitively as possible. In many cases the patient is fully aware of their diagnosis and has not discussed it with their relatives in an attempt to protect them from bad news. Above all it is important to be totally honest. If they ask a question that you do not know the answer to, then say so and offer to find out for them.

Mobile technology

Increasingly, district nurses are embracing mobile technology and moving to a paperless way of working. This means that recorded notes need to be accurate and contemporaneous, to ensure staff visiting afterwards have an up-to-date picture of events and care given. All assessments such as care plans, Malnutrition Universal Screening Tool (MUST) and Waterlow records may be available online with the only paperwork in a patient's home being drug authorisation charts, catheter paperwork, syringe pump charts and end-of-life paperwork.

This way of working presents its own set of challenges. Connectivity can be a problem, particularly in rural areas, as can the device issued to the nurse. Some areas have small tablets or smartphones, whereas other areas may have cumbersome laptops. These devices can also be seen as a barrier to communication within a patient's house: some patients may be suspicious of them and wonder what we are writing, whilst others feel inhibited by them. Whilst modern technology can be a wonderful tool it can also become a barrier to communication.

Much communication is still either face to face or via mobile phones and this is particularly so with other members of the multidisciplinary team such as GPs, Macmillan Nurses and social services. District nurses care for a hugely diverse community and good communication skills develop over time with experience, self-awareness and reflection.

10 Initial assessment and collaborative working

Georgina Newbury, QN and Jayne Foley, QN

Figure 10.1   The multidisciplinary team.

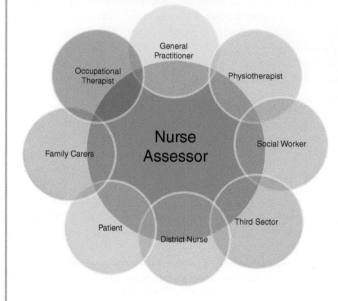

- General Practitioner
- Occupational Therapist
- Physiotherapist
- Family Carers
- **Nurse Assessor**
- Social Worker
- Patient
- District Nurse
- Third Sector

Figure 10.2   A district nurse visits a man living at home with complex healthcare needs.

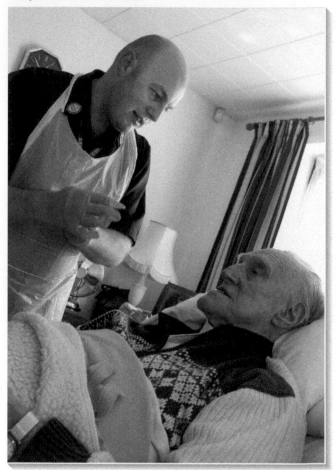

District Nursing at a Glance, First Edition. Edited by Matthew Bradby.
© 2022 John Wiley & Sons Ltd. Published 2022 by John Wiley & Sons Ltd.

The multidisciplinary team

The face of traditional community teams has changed over the past 5–10 years to meet the policy agenda of delivering care nearer to the patient's home. Enabling frail elderly patients and those with complex care needs to remain in their own homes presents challenges. These challenges can only be met by using the combined individual skills of the inter-professional team in a cohesive manner. How the teams look may differ within the four countries of the UK, but their underlying principles remain the same.

Inter-professional teams (or multidisciplinary teams) often work best when physically based within the same location, allowing for easier communication and an appreciation of each other's roles. These teams are made up of doctors, nurses, allied health professionals, social care services and, importantly but sometimes overlooked, the third sector of voluntary services, which can provide extra support and expertise. As with all team working, role dynamics are crucial to success. Traditionally, doctors have often been seen as the leaders of inter-professional teams; however, within the community, district nurses are increasingly taking the leadership role as the key coordinators of care. They will be the first health professional within the team to meet with the patient with initial referrals coming from GPs, families and carers or other district nursing teams. Their responsibility is then to ensure that the right team members are informed of the patient's needs and involved in planning their care in the most efficient, safe and appropriate manner.

Assessment and referral

Patients with complex and enduring health problems are increasing in number and the degree of frailty within the ageing population is apparent to all health professionals. District nurses may well have the required advanced assessment skills, but the size of general caseloads makes managing the complexities of inter-professional referrals time-consuming and this runs the risk of being uncoordinated. District nurses must have a strong understanding of their local population's health needs, including people who may be socially marginalised.

Inter-professional working is very rewarding for professionals working within these teams. They are a cohesive working group with clear goals for excellent patient care. Nurses work particularly well within such teams; however the skills required are at an advanced level. Nurses who are involved in the complex assessment process will have undertaken further education, often holding a recognised specialist practice qualification. A true understanding of community care provision is imperative and a working knowledge of how ongoing services are provided helps with complex decision-making. Nurses without this knowledge may well possess excellent assessment skills, but may be more reliant on the input of secondary care.

Referrals to allied health professionals, including occupational therapists, physiotherapists, or speech and language therapists, will ensure that the patient's ability to remain safely within their own home is considered from every angle (Figure 10.1). The medical registrar or consultant provides the necessary specialist intervention and social care can be organised to provide vital support with daily living. These packages are often provided as a short-term intervention, giving the social worker time to assess and organise an ongoing package of care. This integrated approach has proven vital in managing patients discharged to the community after an admission for Covid-19.

Patients are often initially referred to district nursing services when they are at risk of falling at home. The nurse needs to be able to undertake a holistic assessment using a range of assessment tools. The key elements of an assessment in this situation will involve the nurse carrying out a full physical, psychological, social and environmental assessment. Their role then is to assess, plan and implement care in a personalised manner. Computer systems are crucial to the success of high-quality care delivery and these continue to develop, with better communication referral packages being introduced into the health system. Access to a patient's past medical history and prescription drugs is imperative within the initial assessment phase. Timely care can only be provided when information can be shared instantly.

Nurses undertaking highly specialist initial assessment roles can subsequently miss the opportunity to 'nurse', as once the intense period of the assessment is over, any ongoing nursing care will be referred on to the district nursing team within the locality. However, other professionals such as the physiotherapist and occupational therapist may well have ongoing interaction with the patient, developing longer therapeutic relationships (Figure 10.2).

The third sector and carers

Working with the third sector has added to the diversity and richness of services, with befriending schemes – Age UK and the British Red Cross for example – being crucial within a true inter-professional team. They can provide the small but important services that may fall outside the remit of either health or social services. They are also able to support carers, who themselves may be elderly and may, possibly, have previously been reliant on the person who has now become the patient. Carers, as is increasingly well understood, are the vital backbone of personal social care within the UK; however, many of them are still not recognised for the important role they provide within the community.

Good inter-professional working can assist in meeting NHS targets, but it also keeps patients in their own homes for longer, with ongoing care being passed back to their GP and local district nursing team after a crisis has been averted.

11 Safer caseloads: service planning and caseload allocation

Celine Grundy, QN, Helen Wheeler, Paula Wood, QN, and Rachel Hogan, QN

Figure 11.1   Safe caseload management methods and tools. Source: National Quality Board (2018).

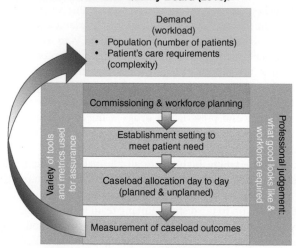

Demand
(workload)
- Population (number of patients)
- Patient's care requirements (complexity)

Variety of tools and metrics used for assurance

Commissioning & workforce planning

↓

Establishment setting to meet patient need

↓

Caseload allocation day to day (planned & unplanned)

↓

Measurement of caseload outcomes

Professional judgement: what good looks like & workforce required

Box 11.2   Key factors for work allocation.

- Patient need
- Complexity of care needed
- Capacity of own and other health and social care services
- Use of technology to support allocation
- Local geographical factors, such as housing and travel time
- Priority of patients
- Skills and knowledge of the team

Box 11.1   Recommendations to support nurse staffing in the district nursing service.

1 Organisations should work together locally, to define safety in the context of district nursing and agree a suite of metrics to provide assurance of safety and quality across the system.
2 Include metrics regarding: patient outcomes, patient safety, patient experience, staff experience with system-wide measures. Standardise collection and monitoring of metrics.
3 Plan the multi-professional workforce to provide safe caseload management around the agreed definitions of safety and quality.
4 Use technology to support remote monitoring and a more agile workforce.
5 Use an evidence-informed decision support tool, triangulated with professional judgement and comparison with relevant peers.
6 Undertake an annual strategic staffing review of all healthcare professional groups.
7 Review a comprehensive staffing report after six months to ensure workforce plans are still appropriate.
8 Review a local dashboard of quality indicators to support decision-making on a monthly basis.
9 Review local recruitment and retention priorities regularly and maximise flexible employment options and efficient deployment of staff.
10 Introduce a process to determine additional uplift requirements based on the needs of patients and local demography.
11 Introduce an escalation process in case staffing does not deliver the outcomes identified in the appropriate plan.
12 Respond to changing patient requirements and new ways of working/ new care models.

Source: National Quality Board (2018).

Figure 11.2   Nine characteristics of good-quality care in district nursing. Source: Maybin et al. (2016).

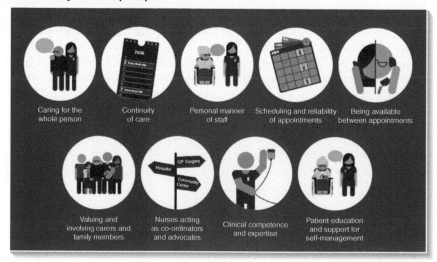

Caring for the whole person

Continuity of care

Personal manner of staff

Scheduling and reliability of appointments

Being available between appointments

Valuing and involving carers and family members

Nurses acting as co-ordinators and advocates

Clinical competence and expertise

Patient education and support for self-management

Box 11.3   Additional key factors for work allocation.

- Right time, right place, right skills (National Quality Board, 2016)
- Dependency needs of the patient (Midlands Partnership Foundation Trust, 2018)
- Escalation policy – for guidance (Midlands Partnership Foundation Trust, 2018)
- Unplanned care and rescheduled visit guidance (Midlands Partnership Foundation Trust, 2018)

District Nursing at a Glance, First Edition. Edited by Matthew Bradby.
© 2022 John Wiley & Sons Ltd. Published 2022 by John Wiley & Sons Ltd.

Patient demand

In the UK – as in many European countries – there is an ageing population with increasing frailty and complexity of need and consequently greater dependence on health and social care services. Figures show that the number of people in the UK aged over 80 is now over three million and this number is projected to double by 2030. This requires a structured approach to the allocation of workload within district nursing services, which offer vital support to many people in this age range. The Covid-19 pandemic has also affected the older population far more severely than the population as a whole, putting additional strain on health services.

The National Institute for Health and Care Excellence (NICE) published guidance in 2014 that sets out evidence-based guidance for staff-to-patient ratios in adult acute settings. Subsequently, many studies have tried to develop similar guidance for community nursing staffing levels.

Safer caseloads

Professor Alison Leary, Professor of Healthcare and Workforce Modelling at London South Bank University and Director of the QNI International Community Nursing Observatory (ICNO), states that, 'District Nursing is easily the most complex nursing work I have ever observed' (Queen's Nursing Institute, 2014). There are multiple variables which impact upon the complexity of the care provided that are often unpredictable and therefore difficult to measure, which makes safe staffing in community nursing very difficult to define. The Queen's Nursing Institute's view is that it is usually more appropriate to speak of 'safer caseloads' rather than 'staff-to-patient ratios' in attempting to determine the workforce needs in the community.

District nurses often describe their service as acting like a sponge; that is, under most circumstances district nursing services do not refuse referrals, but find ways of visiting all patients in need. As such, the allocation of district nursing work is becoming increasingly challenging, not only because of the number of patients needing care but also due to the complexity of their needs. The demand has to be balanced with ensuring that the service is financially and operationally sustainable.

The process of caseload allocation

The process of work allocation involves the planning, organisation, coordination and delegation of visits to patients and other work required (Bain and Baguley, 2012) and although there have been a number of models developed to assist nurses with this process, often these will only meet local requirements. Work commissioned by NHS England (NHSE/QNI, 2014) has identified that several allocation systems are available, but most of these were developed around local requirements and were operational in nature, focusing on scheduling, caseload allocation or validation and assurance of performance data.

In determining safe caseloads in the community, many factors must be considered. First, the skill mix of the community nursing teams must be reviewed. Second, the capacity of community nursing teams must be addressed and there are multiple issues that impact upon their efficiency and effectiveness. In order to collate the information required to determine what safe caseloads might look like, commissioners and service planners utilise software tools. However, currently not all tools that are in use across the NHS cover all metrics required. There are multiple software platforms in use across the NHS, and in many cases their reliability and validity has yet to be evidenced.

The National Quality Board (2018) has reviewed multiple factors that influence safe caseloads. This document has been designed to break down those influencing factors to evaluate the evidence base leading to a series of recommendations (Box 11.1). Allocation of work forms part of caseload management alongside service planning and cannot be treated in isolation. This is illustrated in Figure 11.1 (National Quality Board, 2018). Boxes 11.2 and 11.3 also list some key factors that need to be considered when allocating workload. In addition to the considerations in Box 11.1, there is a need to ensure that the caseloads are efficient, as a result of being robustly reviewed (Grundy and Wheeler, 2018).

Conclusion

The King's Fund (2016) has recommended that more robust national data on capacity and demand in district nursing services is needed, in order that the gaps in capacity and demand can be addressed. The King's Fund identified nine characteristics of good-quality care in district nursing (Figure 11.2 and Box 11.2). This should provide some guidance to both commissioners and front line staff when considering how best to manage caseloads to ensure safe and effective care.

Of all the considerations to be taken into account when allocating workload, having an adequate workforce must be a priority. In the absence of a robust dependency classification system, allocation of team members to deliver care in patients' homes and communities relies on professional judgement. Although there may be software systems to support allocation, it is often much more complex than simply allocating a time slot for a particular activity. Given the many variables affecting nursing in the community setting, the issue of safer caseloads is an ongoing project. The Specialist Practitioner Qualification prepares nurses to lead and manage caseloads effectively and therefore it is vital that these programmes continue to be delivered.

Skill mix in the community

Ann Cubbin, QN

Figure 12.1   An illustration of nurses in the community, from an animated film made by the Queen's Nursing Institute and Hallam Medical in 2021 to celebrate the World Health Organization Year of the Nurse and the Midwife.

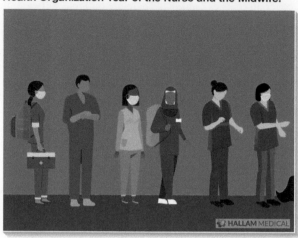

Figure 12.2   An illustration of members of a multidisciplinary healthcare team, from the QNI/Hallam animated film. To see the full film, go to: https://vimeo.com/587749712

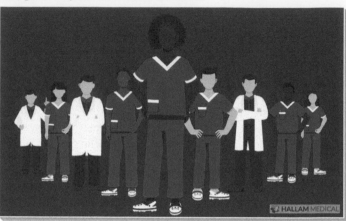

Figure 12.3   Members of a multidisciplinary community healthcare team assess a man in a community setting.

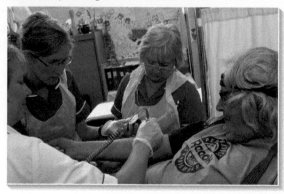

Figure 12.4   Staff members of a community healthcare organisation in the UK wearing personal protective equipment during the Covid-19 pandemic.

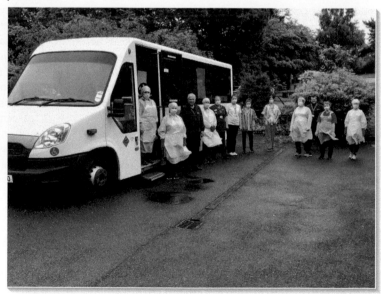

District Nursing at a Glance, First Edition. Edited by Matthew Bradby.
© 2022 John Wiley & Sons Ltd. Published 2022 by John Wiley & Sons Ltd.

All community nursing teams will have a mix of registered nurses and healthcare assistants, but the structure of community teams can vary immensely. Many community teams are constantly changing to maximise efficiency while reducing staff costs, and this has resulted in a reduction of qualified nurses, especially district nurses and an increase in the number of healthcare assistants. To understand skill mix within community nursing teams you need to understand the roles of the individuals within the team (Figure 12.1).

Healthcare assistant

Healthcare assistants (HCAs) are able to undertake a well-defined or routine clinical or non-clinical duty. These tasks have been delegated to them by a registered practitioner, within the limits of their knowledge, skills and competency. They work within standard procedures, protocols and systems but have been provided with additional skills to work autonomously. They are expected to respond to the patients' needs appropriately and report back to the registered practitioner. They are not expected to make changes to the treatment or undertake any assessments or work outside of their ability.

This is not to say they are not experts in some areas of practice (e.g. phlebotomy) and if so they are expected to support the development of this skill in others. A more experienced HCA is expected to make non-complex decisions in additional to the above and report these back, to aid patient care evaluations. They are also in a position to support students, new members of staff and social care staff in an educational capacity.

Assistant practitioner/associate practitioner

This is a relatively new role that is gaining prominence. Assistant practitioners have been provided with a strong educational base in order for them to undertake additional activities beyond those of a HCA. They have a level of autonomy regarding patient care within their recognised level of competency. They may be expected to undertake the allocation of work to HCAs and to supervise the development of student nurses and HCAs.

Nursing associate

Nursing associates focus on patient care, bridging the gap between HCAs and qualified nurses. The focus is on clinical duties and taking more of a lead in decision-making when delivering care. Training is via a 2-year apprenticeship, leading to a foundation degree with the potential to continue training to become a registered nurse. The education and training process has both academic assessments and set standards of proficiency. These proficiencies include medicine management (within set boundaries), invasive and non-invasive procedures such as the insertion of a cannula or urinary catheter, supervised by a registered nurse or another registered professional.

Community staff nurse

This role requires the consolidation of registrant competencies within a community setting where having the confidence, knowledge and skills to make autonomous clinical decisions is paramount to ensuring patients' health and wellbeing. They work without direct supervision in a variety of settings to provide nursing care to patients, who will present with a wide range of healthcare needs. They need to have excellent interpersonal and communication skills to support the patients and to act as advocates on their behalf to other healthcare or social care providers. They actively engage in quality assurance processes and service development, acting as a mentor to less qualified staff and students. More experienced community staff nurses are encouraged to gain additional skills and may act as a team expert or champion in a specific disease pathway, such as dementia or end-of-life care. Many senior community staff nurses are also nurse prescribers from a limited formulary (Figure 12.2).

District nurse

A district nurse has undertaken an additional programme of study and is recorded as a district nurse on the NMC register. They are able to make clinical decisions and evaluations of complex healthcare needs, undertaking the assessments of both new and existing patients. They are actively involved in clinical and team development and will act as a source of expert knowledge and support. They have management responsibilities and can be responsible for the quality of care delivery for a defined caseload. They are the named key worker in end-of-life or complex care (Figure 12.3).

Advanced nurse practitioner

An advanced nurse practitioner has achieved and consolidated at an advanced nursing level, possessing highly specialist knowledge in community nursing. The role may differ across different organisations but the key components of research development, dissemination and implementation along with service quality development and education are fundamental to the role. For an advanced nurse practitioner, patient contact continues to form part of the role but this may evolve into a specialism where they act in a consultancy role for the wider healthcare team.

Conclusion

In addition to the skill constructs within a team there are organisation structures that change the composition of community teams. An 'intermediate care team' is a partnership team of health and social care staff working together to prevent admission or readmission and to facilitate timely hospital discharge. 'Cluster teams' work together to cover a mixed geographical area and are popular in rural areas. They are not affiliated to any one general practice but will support several. Once achieved, a team with a good skill mix works together to provide evidenced based care for patients, and in turn will nurture and support all team members (Figure 12.4).

Nurse prescribing

13

Dianne Hogg, QN

Figure 13.1 District nurse and pharmacist discuss medications.

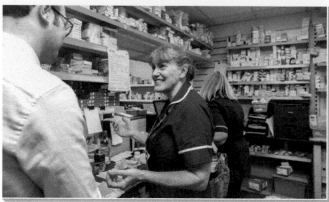

Figure 13.2 Sources of support and information for non-medical prescribers.

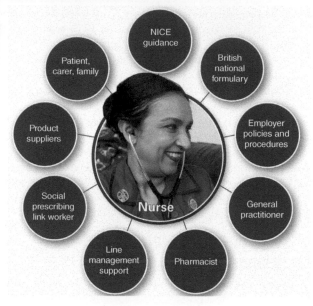

NICE guidance

Patient, carer, family

British national formulary

Product suppliers

Employer policies and procedures

Nurse

Social prescribing link worker

General practitioner

Line management support

Pharmacist

Box 13.1 Sources of information – prescribing.

Royal College of Nursing
- https://www.rcn.org.uk/get-help/rcn-advice/non-medical-prescribers

Misuse of Drugs Regulations 2001
- https://www.legislation.gov.uk/uksi/2001/3998/contents/made

National Institute of Health and Care Excellence
- https://www.nice.org.uk/guidance

British National Formulary
- https://bnf.nice.org.uk/

Nursing and Midwifery Council
- https://www.nmc.org.uk/education/becoming-a-nurse-midwife-nursing-associate/becoming-a-prescriber/

NHS Supply Chain
- https://www.supplychain.nhs.uk/

District Nursing at a Glance, First Edition. Edited by Matthew Bradby.
© 2022 John Wiley & Sons Ltd. Published 2022 by John Wiley & Sons Ltd.

Today, most Nursing and Midwifery Council (NMC)-recorded district nurses are community practitioner nurse prescribers (CPNPs) and many of their community nurse team colleagues have undertaken the stand-alone course (known as V150) to be able to prescribe in the same way. They are able to manage most of their patients' wounds and continence needs without delay or prolonged distress; prescribing at the time and place of contact instead of requesting scripts from other prescribers, such as GPs, with the associated shared accountability complications.

Prescribing by community and district nurses is so much an integral part of day-to-day practice that it would be difficult to envisage the role without it. Hundreds of thousands of products are prescribed annually by CPNPs, theoretically at no additional cost to the NHS – this is replacement prescribing, not additional. In fact, CPNPs are hugely cost-effective:

- In general, the cost for a district nurse to prescribe is much less than that for a GP.
- The district nurse often sees the patient regularly, so will review the prescribing decision on an ongoing basis.
- District nurses tend to prescribe smaller amounts more frequently and can commence treatment very quickly.
- They prescribe only in their areas of competence and repeat prescribing is only possible if the prescriber has seen the patient recently.
- They play a big part in the implementation of wound and continence formularies.

Nurse independent/supplementary prescriber

Some district nurses, through taking a V300 course, have become nurse independent/supplementary prescribers (NISPs) and are able to prescribe from a wide range of medicines, as long as they have adequate competence to do so and their service requires it. NISPs can prescribe similar medicines to those that a CPNP would and may also prescribe other medicines, such as end-of-life medicines and antibiotics (Figure 13.1).

Governance

Organisations are expected to have governance systems and processes in place to support and monitor non-medical prescribing. Non-medical prescribing leads provide the infrastructure and leadership to enable clinical services to select the right candidates to train as prescribers, to consider non-medical prescribing during service redesign; to ensure safe and effective prescribing by monitoring prescribing activity and facilitating ongoing learning; and undertaking scrutiny of personal formularies; and by providing the necessary materials for a prescriber to prescribe (e.g. prescription pads). In some organisations, they provide prescribers with data about their prescribing, which increases a sense of accountability, especially if the data are shared with service leads and commissioners (Figure 13.2).

The future of non-medical prescribing

Non-medical prescribing, particularly by NISPs, involves an adaptable set of competencies, enabling services to develop. Current trends envision a future where district nurses contribute to patient pathways, such as acute care in the home, management of patients with long-term conditions and palliative care. The use of CPNPs will go some way towards enabling fulfilment of this vision, but the implementation of NISPs goes much further, helping to streamline the patient's care pathway and enabling them to live with their condition, rather than being controlled by it.

An example of where this is already happening is where antibiotics are being administered intravenously (IV) to the patient at home. Often the course can be completed orally if the infection responds well, but this usually is not predictable at the start of treatment. If the district nurse is administering the IV antibiotic, making an ongoing assessment of the patient's progress towards recovery, it is a natural progression for the district nurse to prescribe the oral antibiotic – following the pre-defined assessment process and regimen.

The impact of this is set to be much greater as the number of nurse prescribers expands. In 2018, the NMC published 'Future Nurse: Standards of proficiency for registered nurses', which defined the knowledge and skills that registered nurses must demonstrate when caring for people (Nursing and Midwifery Council, 2018c). The standards include proficiencies that enable the nurse to be 'prescribing ready' on qualification to register entry; for example, section 4.17 expects the registered nurse to demonstrate and apply sufficient pharmacology knowledge to have 'the ability to progress to a prescribing qualification following registration'. The entry requirements for post-registration prescribing preparation programmes have changed to reflect these new standards; nurses will need to demonstrate the relevant skills and knowledge to prescribe without waiting for up to 3 years post-registration before application. These changes have the potential to enable more nurses to become prescribers if their roles require it.

Medicines optimisation

Non-medical prescribers are also attuned to the wider aspects of medicines optimisation. An audit undertaken in 2014 by almost 1550 non-medical prescribers in the North West of England (Health Education North West, 2015) included responses from 17 district nurse CPNPs in one organisation who recorded their prescribing-related interventions during 56 patient contacts. The district nurse prescribers reviewed their patient's existing medicines looking for issues related to symptom control, adherence to the medicines regimen, side effects and interactions. The prescribers detected issues that required them to stop certain medicines, adjust the regimen or refer the patient back to the medical prescriber.

One explanation for this wider view on medicines may be the prescribing education pathway: district nurse prescribers are better able to use resources such as the British National Formulary (BNF), national clinical guidance such as that provided by the National Institute for Health and Care Excellence (NICE) and local formulary resources. They will also appreciate the importance of identifying interactions between medicines, contraindications, incorrect doses, etc. They may also feel more confident to discuss prescribing and medicines with the wider healthcare team caring for their patient, having the background and status as a prescriber.

There is no doubt, and the plethora of prescribing activity bears this out, that non-medical prescribing is a valuable tool for district nurses. However, significant investment would be required to increase the number of NISPs in district nursing for the management of more complex long-term conditions. To do so would contribute to the goals of the NHS Long Term Plan and a cost-effective, patient-centred future (Box 13.1).

Medicines management

Dianne Hogg, QN

Figure 14.1 Yellow Card – making medicines safer. Source: MHRA © Crown Copyright, https://yellowcard.mhra.gov.uk/_assets/files/2017-01-27-Yellow-Card-APP-poster.pdf.

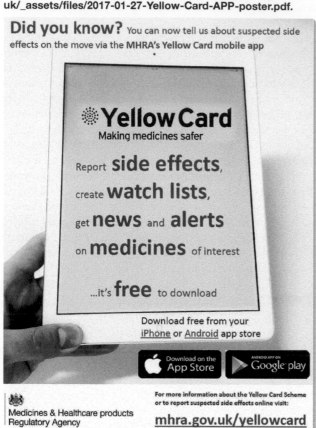

Figure 14.2 A district nurse prepares a needle and syringe for injection.

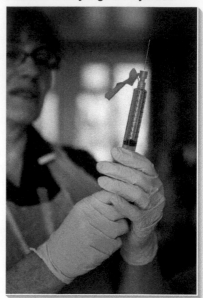

Box 14.1 Six rights of administering medication.

- **Right Person** – People can have very similar, or even the same names. Always make sure you are administering to the right person. For example, check date of birth and medical number.

- **Right Medicine** – Many medicines have similar and complex names. Thoroughly check the name of the drug on the prescription.

- **Right Dose** – Always read the directions and prescribed measure correctly. An underdose is likely to be ineffective. An overdose could cause severe and rapid harm. Wrong doses can also lead to adverse effects in combination drug therapy.

- **Right Route** – Make sure you carefully read how to administer the medication. Getting it wrong can cause harm.

- **Right Time** – Check to see when the medicine was last administered so that medication intervals are as regular as possible.

- **Right to Refuse** – If a person refuses to take their medication, do not try to force them to take it. Document their refusal and any reasons they give, so that appropriate follow up action can be taken, in discussion with colleagues and the person, and in their best interests.

These rights are a useful reference for all staff who may be administering medication.

District Nursing at a Glance, First Edition. Edited by Matthew Bradby.
© 2022 John Wiley & Sons Ltd. Published 2022 by John Wiley & Sons Ltd.

Medicines management and optimisation are the responsibility of every member of the community nursing team. The way that medicines and medicinal products are handled, ordered, prescribed, stored and used has an impact on the way that the medicine works in the patient's body and ultimately on the patient's treatment. This has a knock-on effect on resources, including staff time, the patient's recovery and on organisational finance. The medicines bill is the second largest cost to NHS organisations – destruction of medicines that have been incorrectly stored (in a cupboard instead of a fridge, for example) or medicines that have been over-ordered or unused are unnecessary additions to that bill.

This chapter gives an overview of the considerations that district nurses should make when handling medicines in any way. These are principles and not specific detail, as district nursing is an ever-evolving field of practice, but the general principles of medicines optimisation still apply. There is a plethora of resources available online for further detail.

Medicines policies

All healthcare organisations must have appropriate and up-to-date policies and procedures about medicines. These will be based on current medicines legislation, national interpretation and guidance, professional standards and what that organisation will permit – which may be more restrictive than the aforementioned guidelines, but cannot be more permissive. Standards for medicines management may use the term 'in exceptional circumstances' to allow for extremes of practice, for example in remote rural areas. Your organisation may decide that those exceptions should not occur in its geographical area.

Medicines administration

Many aspects of medicines handling are the same wherever the practice is taking place. The six rights of medicines administration apply in any administration scenario and are useful to use as a mental checklist to ensure all considerations are included (Box 14.1). The six rights are:

- Right patient
- Right drug
- Right dose
- Right route
- Right time
- Right to Refuse.

Extra vigilance is necessary in certain circumstances, for example where two similar products are available, or where documentation is complex. It is a sobering to consider that medicines administration errors are frequent; some lead to patient harm, and most are avoidable.

Community-specific issues

The following are just some of the considerations that apply to district nursing practice.

- Transporting medicines between a pharmacy and the patient's home. The journey should be directly from one to the other, and

the medicines should be stored out of sight. Community nurses must never transport cytotoxic medicines or waste in their cars.
- Cool boxes may be needed to transport refrigerated medicines, which should adhere to national standards to maintain the 'cold chain' (i.e. ensure that the medicine is kept at a stable cool temperature).
- Interface issues between care providers (hospitals, community pharmacy, GP, care home, carers, community nursing teams, etc.) can lead to medicines being omitted, not prescribed, or duplicated. Up to 70% of patients experience some problem with their medicines during a change of care setting; adequate checks should take place and communication between all places of care.
- When a patient dies, although the controlled drugs prescribed for end-of-life palliation belonged to the patient when they were alive, they cannot be owned by the patient's beneficiaries. Organisations should have procedures for community nurses to reclaim controlled drugs.
- About 50% of medicines are taken incorrectly (National Institute of Health and Care Excellence estimate). District nurses play a large part in ensuring that patients take their medicines correctly and must take action where there are problems with medicines adherence. They are well placed to understand the reasons and devise solutions.
- District nurses regularly administer medicines over which they have no control of storage. Storage conditions as the manufacturer intended are listed in the 'Summary of Product Characteristics', available online for each licensed medicine and summarised on the leaflet with every product. Nurses working in the community must assure themselves that they are happy that the medicine has been kept suitably, safely and in a clean environment, before giving the medicine.
- In community practice, most medicines are either supplied or administered to patients on prescription or Patient Group Direction (PGD). PGDs can only be used by registered health professionals; users should have training in their use and have read and signed each one and every ensuing update.
- As district nurses often know their patients well or have visited previously, they are in an ideal position to identify suspected adverse drug reactions (ADRs) and report them. For example Nicorandil, used to treat angina, causes skin blistering in some patients and district nurses may be called upon to dress the blisters. This is a serious ADR and should be reported on a Yellow Card via www.mhra.gov.uk/ yellowcard (Figure 14.1). Identifying and reporting ADRs is an important aspect of the district nurse's role, is a Nursing and Midwifery Council (NMC) 'must-do' and contributes to patient safety on a wider scale. For more information and online learning on ADRs and the Yellow Card scheme see https://www.gov.uk/the-yellow-card-scheme-guidance-for-healthcare-professionals.

Handling medicines is one of the most important roles of a district nurse and should be taken very seriously (Figure 14.2). The list above is not exhaustive; the unique situations a district nurse works in brings different challenges, but the points discussed in this chapter will help to reduce risk for both patient and nurse.

Patient documentation

Angela Reed-Fox, QN

Figure 15.1 Writing up clinical notes in a patient's home during a visit. Patient notes can be recorded on paper or increasingly, in electronic format.

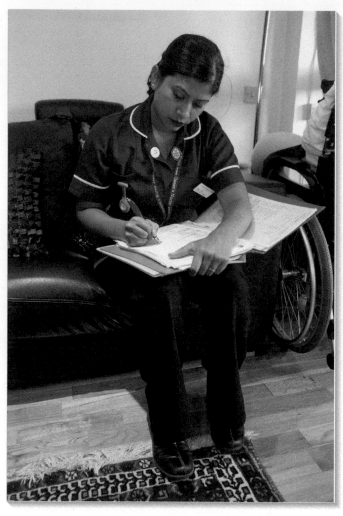

District Nursing at a Glance, First Edition. Edited by Matthew Bradby.
© 2022 John Wiley & Sons Ltd. Published 2022 by John Wiley & Sons Ltd.

Good documentation is an essential part of nursing intervention, and an indispensable component of safe and effective care.

Good documentation improves accountability. It shows how clinical decisions are reached, and it shows care plans and changes in care, as well as the rationale behind these decisions. Good clinical records provide a reliable foundation for the next clinician's consideration of the patient. Accurate, concise and comprehensive records save time, avoid inconsistencies and enable the patient to receive standardised and person-centred care.

Medical records may include a variety of material such as handwritten entries, correspondence between clinicians and patient, lab reports, photographs and imaging records, videos and printouts from monitors, as well as, increasingly, the electronic record.

Essential features of reliable record keeping include:

- Identification of the clinician(s) involved in the intervention – full name and role. Paper records should also be signed. On paper records there may be a signature sheet attached to identify each clinician involved in the patient's care.
- Ensure you are familiar with the relevant documentation policies for your employer/locality.
- Record the date and the time the intervention took place – and the date when the record was entered into the notes if this is different.
- Always write concisely and with clarity, sticking to facts rather than opinion (unless considering differential diagnoses).
- Do not use abbreviations or jargon.
- Do not delete anything from the record. If there is an error, carefully note that this is the case and document a correction with time and date, your name and role.
- Avoid generalisations such as 'appears well' or 'good healing'. Where possible, include a degree of measurement (e.g. 'Wound healed to 30% original size').
- Never chart in advance.
- Be aware of busyness – the time when you can least afford to make a mistake will be the time it is most likely to happen.

If documenting wound care, for example, it is important to ensure that the wound is regularly assessed. This should include size, including width, height and depth, and if possible area as well as condition of the periwound skin, exudate level and consistency, odour, signs of infection, current dressing regime and antibiotic status (including sensitivity), recent swab results and assessment results (including Doppler if necessary), and level and quality of pain/discomfort. How long the wound has been present and, if different, how long it has been treated should also be present in the notes. Previous dressings used and a plan for future care should also all be recorded, and when reassessment should be carried out.

If there are any potential risks or problems, you must document how these have been mitigated. The record should be a reliable source of information passed from one clinician to another; include anything that is relevant or useful.

Written records must be completed in black ink, and be readable when scanned or copied. Corrections can be written in, but must be signed and dated. If information is entered in error, just put one line through and sign and date it. The erroneous text must still be legible. With computerised records, generally the identity of the person making changes will be recorded along with the amendment, but if in doubt, always include your name and role (Figure 15.1).

Patient access

Patients have the right to access their own medical records under the Data Protection Act 2018. Patients are also permitted to register for access to parts of their electronic GP record. Records constitute a legal document and material for audit – perhaps to evaluate care given or to analyse where improvements can and should be made. Good documentation is vital when defending a claim or complaint. If a record is detailed and relevant for continuing care, it is also generally sufficient for legal defence.

It is good practice to involve the patient in their care planning as much as possible. General practices are now offering patients access to aspects of their electronic health record. This enables better patient-centred care as patients are able to check details for themselves, look up test results, and have a reference point before their appointment. This will lead to better-informed patients, in greater control of their health, but clinicians need to ensure that data recorded is accurate, as well as being mindful that notes may be read by the patient. The notes are there for the patient's care and therefore the primary emphasis has to be on passing on the required information to other clinicians involved, but mindfulness of patient access will help to reduce instances of patient misunderstanding or worry.

Each healthcare organisation will have policies on use of medical notes and computers. Do not share passwords or leave unlocked computers unattended. You must ensure patient records are kept securely. Patients should not be discussed in areas where the conversation may be overheard by those not connected with that patient's care. You must consider patient confidentiality at all times.

Documentation is a large and unavoidable part of the nursing role. Care needs to be taken to ensure that patient confidentiality is protected, and that data recorded is accurate, relevant, and detailed enough to progress the patient's care. Good documentation is increasingly a vital part of ensuring patient-centred care. Clinicians need to be mindful of the access patients have to their notes, to minimise the risk of misunderstanding with both colleagues and patients.

16 # Risk management

Mandy McKendry, QN

Figure 16.1 Risk matrix. 1–3 = Low risk; 4–6 = Moderate risk; 8–12 = High risk; 15–25 = Extreme risk. Source: National Patient Safety Agency (2008). *A Risk Matrix for Risk Managers*. London: NPSA.

Consequence	Likelihood				
	1	2	3	4	5
	Rare	Unlikely	Possible	Likely	Almost Certain
5 Catastrophic	5	10	15	20	25
4 Major	4	8	12	16	20
3 Moderate	3	6	9	12	15
2 Minor	2	4	6	8	10
1 Negligible	1	2	3	4	5

Box 16.1 Action plan for risk reduction.

Risk issue	Current risk rating	Required actions	New/target risk rating	Review date
Unsafe environments		All staff members will carry mobile phones		
		All staff members will sign in and out each day		
		The shift coordinator will check this at the start and end of each shift		
		All staff members will leave a documented visit list for clients		
		All staff will have undertaken conflict resolution training		
		All staff will ensure their car registrations are available		
		All staff will risk assess each new referral to determine staff required for visits		
		All staff will ensure colleagues are informed of risks in individuals homes		
		All staff cars/vehicles are maintained in good working order		
		All staff will ensure they have both sat nav and maps for use		
		All staff have contact numbers for the management team should problems occur both in and out of hours.		

N.B. The list of risk reduction actions is not exhaustive and there will be many more. This is for example only.

District Nursing at a Glance, First Edition. Edited by Matthew Bradby.
© 2022 John Wiley & Sons Ltd. Published 2022 by John Wiley & Sons Ltd.

Effective risk management is essential to keep both patients and staff safe within community services; however, a precursor of effective risk management is being risk aware.

All activities within district nursing contain risk, yet within the work environment these risks may not always be managed proactively, in part because clinicians may potentially become desensitised to them and in doing so inadvertently put patients and colleagues at the risk of either minor or major harm, depending on the level of risk. Risk assessment is a systematic and effective method of identifying risks and determining the most cost-effective means to minimise or remove them. It is an essential part of any risk management programme.

In order to manage risk appropriately, a district nurse needs to separate those risks that are unacceptable from those that are tolerable. One should evaluate risk in a consistent manner and work to reduce the level of risk. By considering both the likelihood of the risk occurring and the consequences of that risk in the event of it happening, it is possible to identify a potential risk rating score. Consideration should be given to the fact that often risks will have more than one potential consequence.

In 2020, the Covid-19 pandemic has had a significant impact on the work of district nurses and in particular the risks of treating patients at home, including nursing homes. District nursing services have had to adapt rapidly to the effects of the pandemic in order to minimise the risks to staff, patients, carers and families. All nurses working in the community should ensure they are fully up to date with all guidance issued by their employer and relevant national agencies, for example with regard to the use of personal protective equipment (PPE) and hygiene processes.

Risk scoring or grading

The rating of a given risk can be established using a two-dimensional grid or matrix, with consequence as one axis and likelihood as the other. This allows for a consistent approach to risk scoring (Figure 16.1). The steps to take in scoring and grading risk are as follows:

1 Define the risk(s) explicitly in terms of the adverse consequence(s) that might arise from the risk.
2 Determine the consequence score for the potential adverse outcome(s) relevant to the risk being evaluated.
3 Determine the likelihood score(s) for those adverse outcomes. If possible, score the likelihood by assigning a predicted frequency of occurrence of the adverse outcome. If this is not possible, assign a probability to the adverse outcome occurring within a given time frame, such as the lifetime of a project or a patient care episode. If a numerical probability cannot be determined, use the probability descriptions to determine the most appropriate score.
4 Calculate the risk score by multiplying the consequence by the likelihood: C (consequence) $\times$ L (likelihood) $=$ R (risk score) (National Patient Safety Agency, 2008).

Example

It is often easier for staff to describe a risk using the phrase: 'There is a risk that . . '. This helps staff to keep focused and encourages them to explore all related potential hazards. An example of how this may be undertaken is in the case of lone working.

Risk: Lone working

There is a risk that lone working may result in harm to the staff member due to:

- unsafe environment, for example weather conditions;
- allegations of inappropriate behaviour;
- vehicle breakdown leaving staff member stranded;
- experience of physical or verbal abuse.

This list is not exhaustive and will vary depending on clinical setting and other factors.

Once the hazards or risks have been identified these then need to be individually rated using the risk matrix. It is helpful to record this in a risk log (Box 16.1).

Once the risk rating has been identified it is essential to plan corrective or risk reduction actions, which requires clear documentation and record keeping. It is helpful at this stage to identify what an acceptable or target level of risk would be. This target score helps inform and prioritise the required actions needed to reduce the risks to an acceptable and safe level.

Risk management action plans should be shared with all staff to ensure safe practice throughout the team and the risk assessments should be reviewed at regular intervals to ensure they are proactively monitored and amended as required.

The Department of Health and Social Care recommends that the Boards of NHS organisations should ensure that the effort and resources that are spent on managing risk are proportionate to the risk itself. NHS organisations therefore should have in place efficient assessment processes covering all areas of risk. It is also a legal requirement that all NHS staff actively manage risk.

17 Measuring quality and patient outcomes

Susan Harness, QN

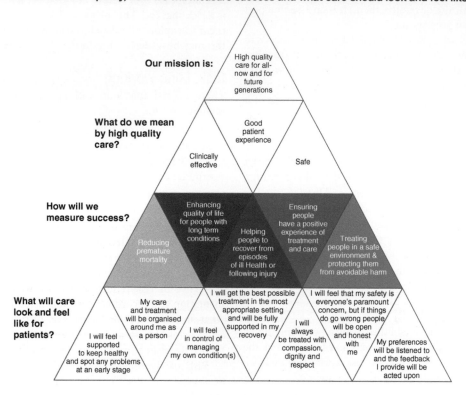

Figure 17.1 Quality of care pyramid. NHS England has developed a pyramid which shows how their mission of ensuring high-quality care for all relates to the definition for quality, how we will measure success and what care should look and feel like for patients.

Our mission is:
High quality care for all- now and for future generations

What do we mean by high quality care?
Good patient experience
Clinically effective
Safe

How will we measure success?
Enhancing quality of life for people with long term conditions
Ensuring people have a positive experience of treatment and care
Reducing premature mortality
Helping people to recover from episodes of ill Health or following injury
Treating people in a safe environment & protecting them from avoidable harm

What will care look and feel like for patients?
My care and treatment will be organised around me as a person
I will get the best possible treatment in the most appropriate setting and will be fully supported in my recovery
I will feel that my safety is everyone's paramount concern, but if things do go wrong people will be open and honest with me
I will feel supported to keep healthy and spot any problems at an early stage
I will feel in control of managing my own condition(s)
I will always be treated with compassion, dignity and respect
My preferences will be listened to and the feedback I provide will be acted upon

Figure 17.2 The NHS Safety Thermometer was developed for the NHS by the NHS as a point-of-care survey instrument. It provides a 'temperature check' on harm that can be used alongside other measures of harm to measure local and system progress in providing a care environment free of harm for patients.

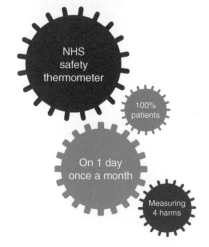

NHS safety thermometer

100% patients

On 1 day once a month

Measuring 4 harms

Defining quality

As health professionals, we all aim to provide care and treatment to our patients that is of high quality. But what do we mean by quality care? How can we measure it?

High-quality care can usually be defined in three parts: clinical effectiveness, safety and patient experience. These three components encompass different perspectives. Patients need treatment that works, meets their needs, that is safe and that is delivered by caring and competent professionals. Clinicians focus on delivering healthcare that is evidence-based and effective in treating patients. Managers and commissioners of services are concerned that quality healthcare is delivered safely, whilst ensuring that it is efficient and cost-effective, and that good outcomes can be demonstrated.

Understanding the patient experience

When talking about how we can improve quality of care, we often take the perspective of a health professional. However, what we as health professionals think patients want or need, may not be the same as what patients actually want. The care that district nurses and their teams deliver needs to have input from patients themselves, and to take account of the views of family members and carers. Patients should be encouraged to share their opinions about the experience of care they received.

Personalised care, as set out the recently published *NHS Long Term Plan* (https://www.longtermplan.nhs.uk/), is now at the heart of healthcare policy and of district nursing care. Personalised care means people have choice and control over the way their care is planned and delivered. It is based on 'what matters' to them and their individual strengths and needs. This happens within a system that makes the most of the expertise, capacity and potential of people, families and communities in delivering better outcomes and experiences. This focus is fundamental if district nurses and their teams are to know where to direct their attention in order to improve services. In 2013, major failings in care were identified in the Francis Report, which recommended that patients need to be listened to, in relation to how we design and deliver services (The Health Foundation, 2015). Understanding patient experience and actively involving patients is key to improving the quality of care. Care must be relevant to the individual and the community to which they belong.

Measuring quality

Patient experience

How district nursing services collect patient views will vary. Services may decide to post a patient satisfaction survey or questionnaire to patients asking them to answer a set of questions. Another tool could be to ask patients to complete an electronic satisfaction survey (which could be online) while care is being delivered. A popular tool is the NHS 'Friends and Family Test' (NHS, 2020), or a text message to service users to ask them to judge their level of patient satisfaction once the care has been delivered (Figure 17.1). From a qualitative perspective, one could decide to interview a number of patients or create a focus group to gain a deeper perspective about how they felt about the care they received and the service as a whole. Nurses may decide to consider the compliments they receive in the form of verbal feedback or thank you cards. Teams could also examine complaints or feedback from patient liaison services. With advances in technology, there are ever greater possibilities to measure patient opinion and to reach out to communities who may in the past have been reluctant to engage with services, for example refugees and asylum seekers.

Care process

Nursing services can also measure the quality of the care process, so that performance can be measured against predefined standards or criteria. An example of this would be to select a topic to audit to determine what area of the care needs to be improved – for example, to audit the standard of documentation within the team against local and national guidelines. Results will identify where the level of documentation is good and meets the set criteria and where it falls short. Other tools to measure quality examine 'significant events'. The intention here is to improve the safety and quality of care by encouraging staff to reflect on the event, learn from it and minimise future risk.

Quality indicators measure a service numerically and help us to understand and compare results with other areas. An example of a quality indicator is the NHS Safety Thermometer (Figure 17.2). This is used throughout England to provide a snapshot of all patients that are seen and identify how many have come to healthcare-associated harm in the care setting. The data collected gives us information so that this can be benchmarked and resources allocated to ensure safe and effective care.

To focus on improving the quality of care that we deliver is a challenge for all health professionals. We need to work with patients to access their views and understand what a good or poor experience feels like from the patient perspective. The range of different outcomes demonstrates the multidimensional nature of quality. However, the overall aim is to implement improvements so that patient outcomes are positive and patients are satisfied with the quality of care delivered to them, both in terms of having a good experience and good outcomes. We also need to respect, involve and empower all staff to challenge existing methods and test new ideas for improving quality, and share a commitment towards a quality agenda for all patients.

18 Caring for yourself in the community setting

Anita Clough, QN and Neesha Oozageer Gunowa, QN

Figure 18.1   Many district nurse visits will be to people living alone.

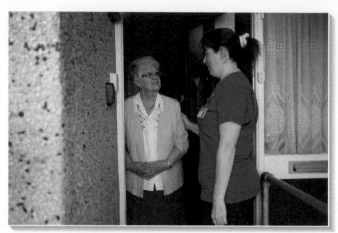

Figure 18.2   Travel by car is usually the most efficient way to reach patients, particularly in rural areas.

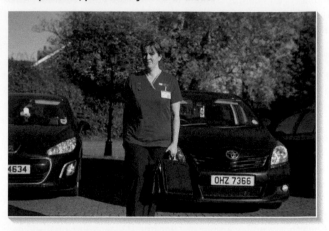

Figure 18.3   Example of a 'Wellbeing Tree' poster for use in a community nursing staff setting. Team members are encouraged to post paper leaves with positive suggestions on to the tree.

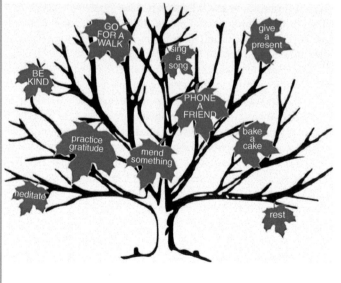

Figure 18.4   Example of a staff 'Wobble Room' poster for use in a community healthcare staff setting. The Wobble Room is a safe space model that has become more widely used during the Covid19 pandemic.

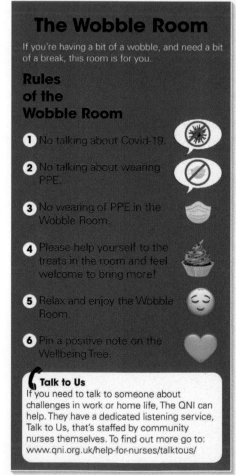

The Wobble Room

If you're having a bit of a wobble, and need a bit of a break, this room is for you.

Rules of the Wobble Room

1. No talking about Covid-19.
2. No talking about wearing PPE.
3. No wearing of PPE in the Wobble Room.
4. Please help yourself to the treats in the room and feel welcome to bring more!
5. Relax and enjoy the Wobble Room.
6. Pin a positive note on the Wellbeing Tree.

Talk to Us
If you need to talk to someone about challenges in work or home life, The QNI can help. They have a dedicated listening service, Talk to Us, that's staffed by community nurses themselves. To find out more go to: www.qni.org.uk/help-for-nurses/talktous/

District Nursing at a Glance, First Edition. Edited by Matthew Bradby.
© 2022 John Wiley & Sons Ltd. Published 2022 by John Wiley & Sons Ltd.

D istrict nurses care for individuals of all ages, having roles in health promotion, prevention of illness, and the care of ill, disabled and dying people. Advocacy, promotion of a safe environment, research, shaping health policy and education are also key roles.

How the district nurse copes with the demands of modern healthcare will have an enormous effect on their ability to coordinate and deliver the care that patients require, while also enabling the nurse to have a fulfilling career and happy work–life balance. The following suggestions are intended to help the district nurse in caring for him- or herself.

Travel

In rural areas, a district nurse can travel for many miles between each patient's home. In cases of severe weather, it may be necessary to cancel or postpone non-urgent patient visits in order to avoid the risk of attempting the journey.

Lone working

District nurses are a vulnerable group of healthcare professionals because they travel to patients' own homes and work mainly alone. When working in isolation, whether it is in the inner city or in a rural area, it is important to consider one's own safety and the safety of colleagues. Most community teams will have a set of criteria for assessing the suitability of home visits for their patients (Figure 18.1).

The employing Trust has a duty of care to its staff and a lone working policy must be in place. The lone working policy will address issues such as how referrals are received. If possible, all new referrals to community nurses should be checked with practice records for any history of mental health problems, substance use, or violence and aggression, both in respect of the patient but also in the household or location. As teams will vary in size, local arrangements should be place to ensure that a colleague can always identify where a community nurse is at any given time. This contact person may be another member of the team or, in the case of small teams, it may be a receptionist in the clinical area to which the nurse is attached. A policy should include a procedure for checking that all staff are safe and accounted for at the end of every shift.

Time management

Using time efficiently is a goal that all healthcare professionals need to strive towards. Particularly in the community, nurses work autonomously and have to plan their day to suit various appointment times within the working day (Figure 18.2). Trusts and healthcare settings use various methods to ensure staff use time in an efficient manner. 'Releasing time to care' is a programme that enables clinicians to identify the amount of time spent in delivering hands-on care and helps them to streamline systems so that less time is spent doing other non-clinical administrative tasks

(NHS England, 2020). Establishing good time management within the work environment enables nurses to plan their day efficiently and make time for a lunch break or personal development. Evidence shows that nurses who are overtired are more likely to cause or make mistakes within the clinical environment, which in turn can lead to stress, which accounts for over one-third of all new incidents of sickness.

Mental wellbeing

With constant pressures on the nursing workforce, tasks and day-to-day activities can at times be strenuous. Competing demands and increased expectations with fewer resources mean that nurses are at times having to compromise. Having to compromise care can be very distressing for a nurse and can lead to mental ill health. It is therefore important to raise concerns early with a manager and discuss them with your team (Figures 18.3 and 18.4).

Clinical supervision

Clinical supervision is an activity of ever-growing importance for nurses in the community setting. Clinical supervision refers to facilitating reflective practice, enabling nurses to question and evaluate their own practice, supporting each other by offering a sounding board and exploring options for coping and developing, both within themselves and for patient care. Clinical supervision can be very effective in empowering practitioners in the community setting, as it provides the opportunity to effectively manage and cope with the demanding situations clinicians face. These situations include working in isolation, emotional involvement with patients and carers, rapid role expansion and increased professional responsibility, dissemination of best practice, continual change within practice settings and patients being discharged with increasingly complex needs.

Physical wellbeing

As well as being mentally draining at times, district nursing can also be physically exhausting, with attendant health and safety risks. Despite all nurses attending mandatory moving and handling training, a quarter of all nurses have taken some time off due to a back injury. Whilst working in a community setting, district nurses will encounter diverse home environments which cater for the needs and preferences of the home owner or occupier, rather than for nursing practice. At times this can result in working in confined spaces with limited movement, for example.

Caring for oneself is one's own responsibility; however, employers also have a legal duty to ensure staff safety and wellbeing. To ensure both staff and employer care for each other in this respect, they must have common values and goals, and clearly share and communicate policies and procedures. It is important that these are established and reinforced through regular one-to-one meetings and a yearly appraisal.

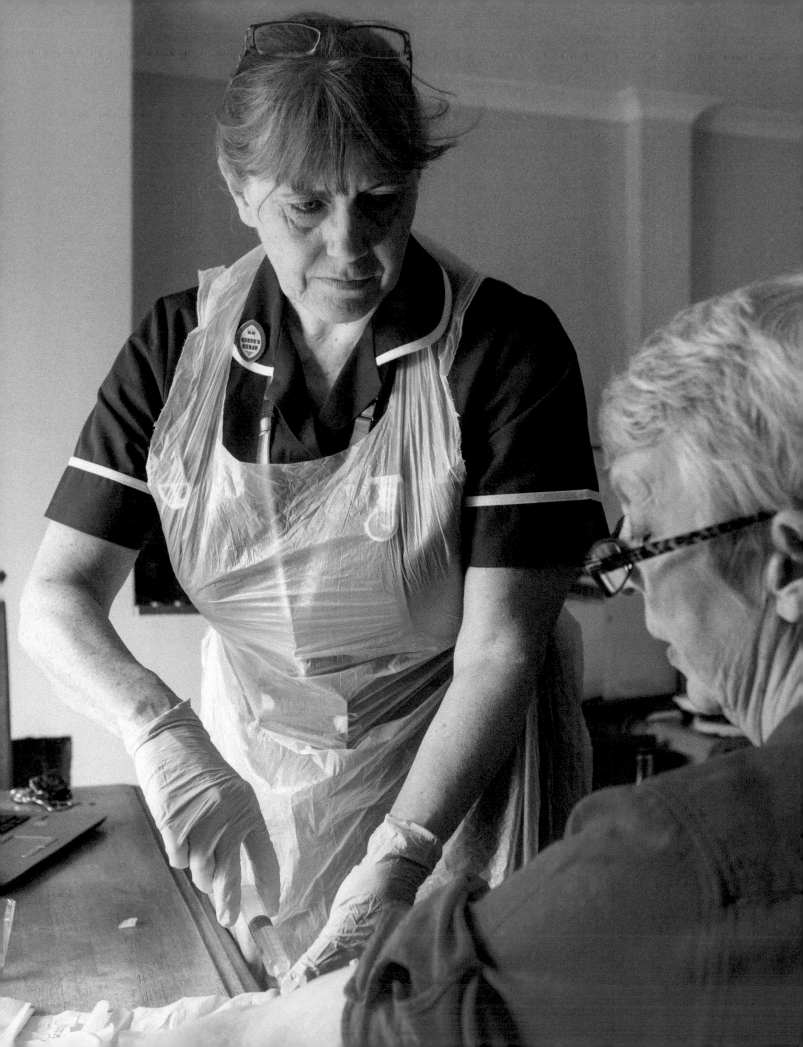

Caring for the whole person in the community

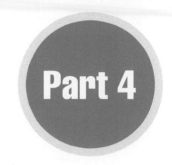

Part 4

Chapters

19 How to make every contact count: health chat

Amanda Huddleston, QN

Figure 19.1 Making every contact count.

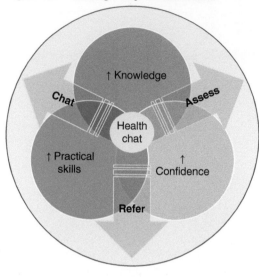

Figure 19.2 Behaviour change interventions mapped to NICE behaviour change: individual approaches. *Source:* https://www.nice.org.uk/Guidence/PH49.

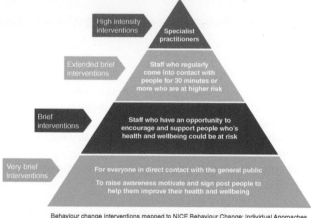

Behaviour change interventions mapped to NICE Behaviour Change: Individual Approaches
https://www.nice.org.uk/Guidance/PH49

Figure 19.3 Example of a Likert Scale for use in healthcare settings.

How would you rate your motivation to increase your level of daily exercise, on a scale of 1 to 10?
(if 1 is not motivated at all, and 10 is very highly motivated).

1	2	3	4	5	6	7	8	9	10

Table 19.1 Some suggested prompts to patient discussion.

Patient interaction	Lifestyle improvement/Topic for discussion
Patient asking about the length of time their wound will take to heal	Smoking reduces effective blood flow and healing
Overweight patient unhappy with poor mobility or joint pain	Losing weight can help relieve these issues
Patient has experienced a fall	Is it due to alcohol? Did they know more activity reduces risk of falls?
Consistent unstable blood sugars	Discuss healthy diet/alcohol intake

District Nursing at a Glance, First Edition. Edited by Matthew Bradby.
© 2022 John Wiley & Sons Ltd. Published 2022 by John Wiley & Sons Ltd.

The Nursing and Midwifery Council (NMC) Code states that nurses have a duty of care to 'work with others to protect and promote the health and wellbeing of those in your care, their families and carers, and the wider community' (Nursing and Midwifery Council, 2016).

Nurse education provides much theory and education regarding health promotion: in practice there are many barriers that mean up to 90% of frontline staff do not feel competent or comfortable discussing individual lifestyle. However, around 90% of patients believe nurses should discuss lifestyle issues that are impacting on their health.

Local primary research by the author regarding these barriers showed that only around 1 in 10 of nurse–patient contacts resulted in a meaningful discussion or intervention. Of these, the majority (85%) were around smoking. Discussions around more sensitive and complex issues such as obesity and alcohol were virtually non-existent.

A review of the evidence and community nursing focus groups showed the following issues to be the main reasons for the practice/theory gap:

- Seeing public health as 'none of my business'
- Fear of alienating patients by causing offence
- Perceived lack of time to resolve issues once highlighted
- Lack of practical knowledge and confidence to support patients
- Confusion regarding terminology such as 'brief intervention'
- Uncertainty as to where to refer/services available.

After extensive testing of the most effective method of improving knowledge and skills, the 'Health Chat' approach was devised and then refined based upon staff feedback. The underpinning principle is to make health promotion, public health and lifestyle advice more fun and less formal. The three key aims of using this approach are to increase frontline staff knowledge of local public health issues, increase confidence in addressing lifestyle issues and provide the skills to have effective conversations with patients.

The 'chat, assess and refer' approach enables nurses to provide quick opportunistic health and lifestyle advice (Figure 19.1). The fundamental skill required is to learn how to quickly assess patient motivation, as this is key to supporting positive change and concordance. Without appropriate motivation, there is little point in dictating or attempting to force someone to change. Instead this is likely to cause damage to the nurse–patient relationship, as nurses feel they are a 'failure', people may be less truthful in the future about their health, and resources, including time, could be wasted, as unmotivated people are not likely to attend referral appointments made for them (Figure 19.2).

So, as nurses, how can we quickly assess motivation? Assessment of motivation needs to be opportunistic but questions should not just be randomly asked. The key in getting an honest answer from the person is to find the right moment or opportunity that is meaningful to them. Some examples of this are listed Table 19.1.

The use of a Likert scale (more commonly known in practice as a 1 to 10 scale) is the fastest and most effective method of assessing motivation. Once the nurse has identified an opportunistic moment and a potential topic related to care, he or she could ask, 'On a scale of 1 to 10, how do you feel about your XXX (insert issue)'. If a low answer is given (typically 4 or less), it is best not to attempt to discuss the issue any further as there is little motivation. At this point the nurse can simply close the discussion with an invitation to revisit the topic any time the patient feels they want to. It is also beneficial to record the discussion (and score) for future reference and so that other staff can use it as a baseline (Figure 19.3).

If the answer is 4 or above, then all you need do is ask the second question: 'On a scale of 1 to 10, how likely are you to want to do anything about it right now?' Again, with a low score, close the discussion with a future option to revisit and record the score and discussion. At this point, the nurse may want to leave a little more information about the issue. Commonly, people need more time and less pressure to make a behaviour change, so this could meet the person's needs. Many staff prefer not to carry around leaflets on different lifestyle issues, so mentioning a useful number, website (e.g. NHS Choices) or signposting patients to a mobile phone app may be enough.

For people who are interested and want to do something about it, it is appropriate to seize the moment. The nurse can give them the details of apps, lifestyle services and local community assets. Better still, have them make an appointment there and then. This is the best approach for two reasons: first, it reconfirms motivation because making the call is the first step; second, it saves time and paperwork for busy community nurses. By using these fast and effective methods the chat, assess and refer model can be delivered in typically less than two minutes.

20 Cultural issues associated with district nursing

Rachel Daly, QN

Figure 20.1 Cultural competence builds on the concepts of cultural awareness and refers to the ability of healthcare providers to apply knowledge and skill appropriately in interactions with clients. Source: Adapted from Srivastava (2007).

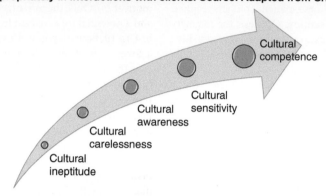

Figure 20.2 Cultural issues in nursing word cloud.

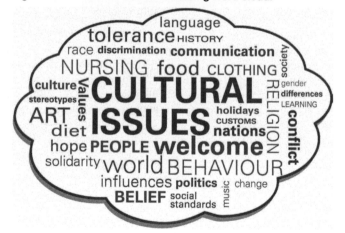

District Nursing at a Glance, First Edition. Edited by Matthew Bradby.
© 2022 John Wiley & Sons Ltd. Published 2022 by John Wiley & Sons Ltd.

This chapter is about encouraging reflection on cultural aspects of practice that might challenge you and your personal values in your professional capacity. In your practice, you should feel confident that you are able to treat people from all cultures in a way that affirms their worth and preserves their dignity.

Culture and ethnicity

Culture is an important means by which people may identify with a larger group; it involves the awareness of shared origins and traditions, and characteristics of a human group relating to racial, ethnic, religious, linguistic and other traits in common. A person's cultural identity may shape their health and wellbeing through their beliefs, values and behaviours.

Whilst culture and ethnicity may be linked, they may equally exist independently of one another and we should never make assumptions about a person's culture based on their ethnicity, religion, nationality, appearance, age or other feature. Definitions of ethnicity suggest that it relates specifically to the classification of humankind, especially on the basis of racial characteristics, but whilst they often overlap, culture and ethnicity are different.

Diversity and personal values

The first weeks of nurse training stress the importance of being non-judgemental, and this is a key theme of nurse education. However, we all make judgements all the time, consciously and subconsciously. It may be useful to reflect on assumptions that we make, based upon an individual's appearance, behaviour or ethnicity. Why have these assumptions been reached? Reflecting on these assumptions might help us to understand our own cultural values and any existing unconscious biases and our cultural competence (Figure 20.1).

Research has identified that health and social care access can be dramatically restricted due to unwitting assumptions based largely upon culture and ethnicity, among other factors (Quickfall, 2004). You may have difficulty aligning some cultures to your own personal values and belief systems; similarly, patients and their families will have a cultural basis for their interactions with you (Figure 20.2). If this is an issue it is likely to be more apparent in the community, because when you enter a person's home or community you may be immersed in their culture and this could cause discomfort, for example with communication problems.

Have you ever considered whether this is an issue that might affect you or make you uncomfortable? Acknowledging cultural challenges to yourself, your mentor and your manager should be seen as positive. There is recognition in research and in local and national policy of the need for adequate support systems in healthcare for both staff and patients, which enable and encourage cultural awareness and understanding (Applebaum, 2017; NHS England, 2017; NHS, 2019a). Cultural self-awareness can enable us to recognise and challenge unconscious bias or prejudice that reinforces inequalities that exist in communities and is the first step towards genuine cultural competence.

Reflecting on the 'micro-cultures' that exist within your own family and community may highlight how readily you adapt to the norms within the cultures around you. A culturally competent nurse recognises different cultural perspectives and has the skills to use his or her knowledge effectively in cross-cultural situations, recognising each person as an individual at the centre of, and a partner in, their own care.

The culture of district nursing

District nursing is different from hospital nursing and that must be taken into account when exploring cultural issues related to nursing in the community. District nursing offers more freedom to work in partnership with patients and other professionals in a person-centred way, which recognises the importance of all elements of a patient's wellbeing. In a hospital setting, this may be more difficult to achieve. In the community, the nurse plans, facilitates, coordinates and delivers care in partnership with the patient and their family in a longer term way that recognises and respects the culture of individuals, their family and their wider community.

Reflection on this culture shift could help nurses moving from the hospital to the community sector. In the community, patients and their family carers are in control; care plans and packages are tailored to suit people's individual requirements, environment and circumstances. For the nurse this takes a level of confidence, skill and competence beyond simply understanding clinical efficacy and therapeutic intent; it requires enhanced communication and understanding of an individual, their nursing and medical needs, personal values and desires in addition to the core nursing values.

Visible leadership is also essential to the creation of an effective and supportive culture in nursing; that is, a culture of valuing individuals (patients, carers, families and staff) that is safe and encourages concerns to be raised. There should be regular opportunities for staff to reflect on their work, explore issues, analyse problems and share best practice.

Because every patient and staff member is an individual with a unique personal history, belief system and communication style, assumptions should never be made about someone based upon ethnicity, race, religion, age, sex, gender, ability or other relevant characteristic. Cultural competence is an important skill for health and social care staff, who deal daily with a richly diverse population in need of support. It involves awareness and sensitivity to different cultures and the ability to treat people from all cultures in a way that affirms their worth and preserves their dignity.

More information about protected characteristics under the Equality Act 2010 can be accessed at https://www.gov.uk/discrimination-your-rights

21 Social isolation and loneliness

Annie Darby, QN

Figure 21.1   Maslow's hierarchy of needs.

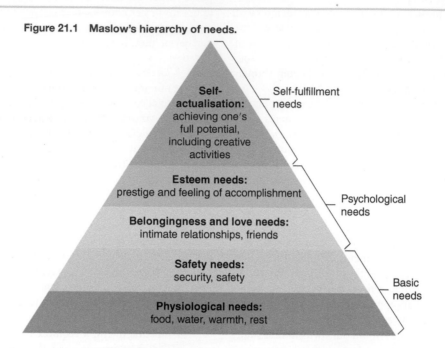

Self-fulfillment needs

Self-actualisation: achieving one's full potential, including creative activities

Esteem needs: prestige and feeling of accomplishment

Psychological needs

Belongingness and love needs: intimate relationships, friends

Safety needs: security, safety

Basic needs

Physiological needs: food, water, warmth, rest

Figure 21.2   Nurse at a homeless health clinic.

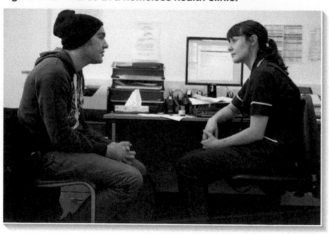

Figure 21.3   Nurse examines feet of a person at a homeless shelter.

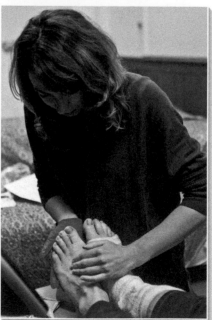

District Nursing at a Glance, First Edition. Edited by Matthew Bradby.
© 2022 John Wiley & Sons Ltd. Published 2022 by John Wiley & Sons Ltd.

The term 'social isolation' often conjures up images of people experiencing homelessness and older people, but it can affect all individuals at all stages and from all walks of life.

Social isolation can be due to a relatively sudden event, caused by bereavement or relocation, or a condition that lasts years. It can affect all areas of a person's life. Someone who is socially isolated will usually not have trusted individuals to turn to at times of illness and crisis, and they may lose the ability and confidence to interact with other people in a positive way. People who are socially isolated are sometimes dismissed as being 'inadequate' but the reality is more complex. If there is little social interaction, then there is no one to measure your behaviour against. Some, though not all, individuals who are socially isolated can present as challenging, which then deepens their isolation.

Social isolation has a corrosive effect on health and how an individual meets their own health needs. Negotiating your way around health and social care systems, including the NHS, can be daunting. Health literacy is a term to describe how competent and confident you are in using services. How informed and health literate you are will equate to how successful you are at accessing the services you are entitled to. It often depends on a person having a degree of literacy and numeracy, and the confidence to attend appointments on time, talk to health professionals and engage with treatment plans. People who are socially isolated often have low levels of health literacy.

Maslow's hierarchy of needs (Figure 21.1) still remains one of the most influential theories relating to the varying needs human beings require if they are to reach their full potential. Central to Maslow's theory is that humans require the following needs to be met: physiological needs, safety and security, love, belonging and esteem. Only if these are met, will humans 'self-actualise'. Put simply, it means that only then will a human be able to accomplish all that they wish to do.

Maslow was very specific about humans needing social contact and a sense of belonging among their social group. If people are deprived of this they become anxious, lonely and depressed. Human beings thrive on friendship, kinship and having a strong social support network: relationships matter and the lack of them can frequently lead to poor health and wellbeing. Having friends, being in a long-term relationship, belonging to clubs and societies all have significant health protection factors.

Social isolation may have consequential effects on all aspects of health. Physical health can suffer through factors associated with social isolation, such as malnutrition, which may exacerbate pre-existing physical health issues. For most people, eating a meal is a socially rewarding event, but a socially isolated person may avoid food shopping and will eat alone. Lack of exercise is another common problem, as someone isolated and alone will often not have any reason to participate in exercise.

As mentioned, anyone can become socially isolated, but certain people are more prone to it. Precipitating factors include mental illness, substance misuse, homelessness, migration or refugee status, and learning difficulties. The elderly are particularly at risk; they may have been bereaved, have no family relationships, or lack the confidence to engage in social activities (Figure 21.2).

Homelessness can take many forms: it is not simply the stereotypical image of rough sleepers whose health is impacted by lack of housing. Many people 'sofa surf', commonly spending a night at a friend's house, then a night in a hostel, interspersed with periods sleeping rough on the streets. As a result they are at risk of many health problems. They go through situations of physical and social isolation, followed by periods of close human contact. An example is those who attend homeless shelters; they receive food, warmth and, in some cases, access to medical treatment, but they may also be exposed to people with tuberculosis and respiratory viruses such as influenza. Their weakened immune system and overall poor state of health not only makes them more susceptible to acquiring infections, but also gives them a slower recovery time and risks exacerbation of pre-existing diseases (Figure 21.3).

For those sleeping on the streets, exposure to the elements will have a negative effect on their health, especially in regard to respiratory, cardiovascular and endocrine disease. The exposure to infectious diseases and the constant threat of violence makes them extremely vulnerable. There is often a strong correlation between homelessness and sexual exploitation, among both men and women. The offer of accommodation to a young homeless person will appear attractive, and may be the start of a spiral downwards into sexual exploitation. This has a damaging effect on psychological wellbeing, especially self-esteem. It also has a detrimental effect on physical and sexual health. Those who are subject to sexual exploitation are frequently exposed to physical assaults and intimidation. They are also at high risk of contracting sexually transmitted infections such as chlamydia and HIV; there is also a strong correlation with illegal drug use.

Social isolation has a detrimental effect on all aspects of health: physical, psychological, sexual and emotional. District nurses must be aware of, and take account of, social isolation in the care and treatment of their patients in the community.

The Queen's Nursing Institute operates a Homeless and Inclusion Health Programme, offering a range of online resources for nurses working with marginalised people. For more information go to: https://www.qni.org.uk/nursing-in-the-community/homeless-health-programme/. For more information about the work of specialist Homeless Health Nurses, see Chapter 71.

Health inequalities and engaging vulnerable groups

Annie Darby, QN

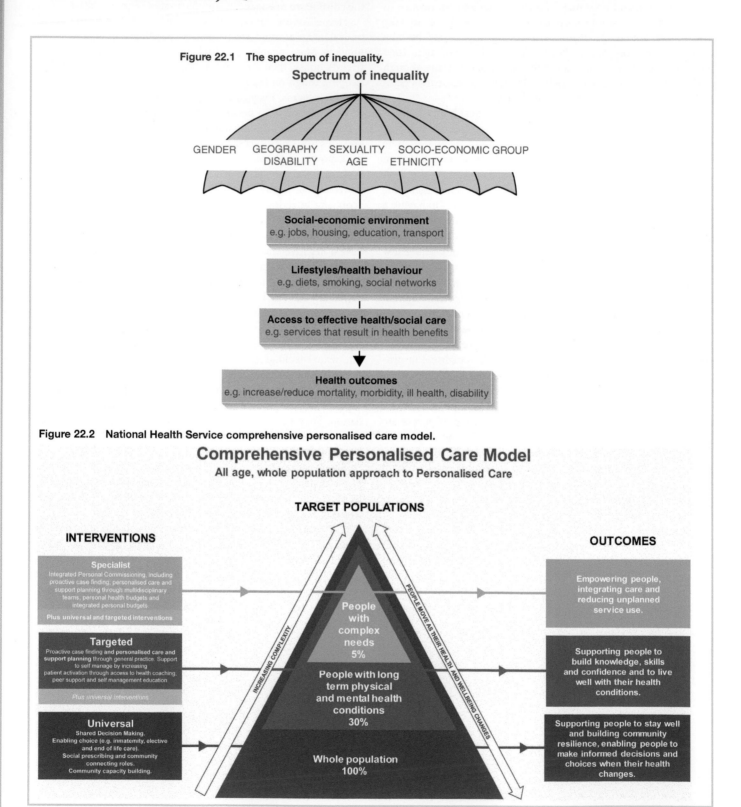

Figure 22.1 The spectrum of inequality.

Spectrum of inequality

GENDER   GEOGRAPHY   SEXUALITY   SOCIO-ECONOMIC GROUP
            DISABILITY   AGE   ETHNICITY

Social-economic environment
e.g. jobs, housing, education, transport

Lifestyles/health behaviour
e.g. diets, smoking, social networks

Access to effective health/social care
e.g. services that result in health benefits

Health outcomes
e.g. increase/reduce mortality, morbidity, ill health, disability

Figure 22.2 National Health Service comprehensive personalised care model.

Comprehensive Personalised Care Model
All age, whole population approach to Personalised Care

TARGET POPULATIONS

INTERVENTIONS

Specialist
Integrated Personal Commissioning, including proactive case finding; personalised care and support planning through multidisciplinary teams; personal health budgets and integrated personal budgets.

Plus universal and targeted interventions

Targeted
Proactive case finding and personalised care and support planning through general practice. Support to self manage by increasing patient activation through access to health coaching, peer support and self management education.

Plus universal interventions

Universal
Shared Decision Making.
Enabling choice (e.g. in maternity, elective and end of life care).
Social prescribing and community connecting roles.
Community capacity building.

INCREASING COMPLEXITY

People with complex needs 5%

People with long term physical and mental health conditions 30%

Whole population 100%

PEOPLE MOVE AS THEIR HEALTH AND WELLBEING CHANGES

OUTCOMES

Empowering people, integrating care and reducing unplanned service use.

Supporting people to build knowledge, skills and confidence and to live well with their health conditions.

Supporting people to stay well and building community resilience, enabling people to make informed decisions and choices when their health changes.

District Nursing at a Glance, First Edition. Edited by Matthew Bradby.
© 2022 John Wiley & Sons Ltd. Published 2022 by John Wiley & Sons Ltd.

'Health inequalities' is a phrase that is used liberally by the media and health and social care workers to explain why some groups in the population fare worse in terms of morbidity and mortality than others. Reducing health inequalities has long been seen as a driving force for the NHS and public health bodies as the definitive proof of how health is improving; however, like most concepts, it is complex. There are many causes of health inequalities, and few are directly related to healthcare provision.

The Marmot Review of 2010 is the most influential report relating to health inequalities in the UK, and it clearly identified that health inequalities are inextricably linked to social justice. The lower a person's social position, the worse their health outcomes are likely to be. Health inequalities cannot be attributed simply to genes, unhealthy behaviour, or difficulties in access to medical care, important as those factors may be. There is often a tendency to apportion 'blame' to individuals and groups, but the reality is far more complex.

It is essential that when talking about health inequalities we encompass all aspects of health, including physical, mental and emotional. We also need to examine the concept of 'wellbeing'. Someone can have a debilitating illness, but enjoy a fulfilling life; likewise an individual may appear to be in good physical health but lack the aspiration and motivation to attain their full potential.

Social and economic inequalities underpin the 'determinants' of health: the range of interacting factors that shape health and wellbeing. These include: material circumstances such as housing; general standard of living; the social environment, which is often the physical neighbourhood someone lives in and their support structure; psychosocial factors; behaviours; and biological factors. Climate change, for example, has a significant effect on health inequalities, adversely affecting food and water supply and air quality. Other factors are social position, education, occupation, income, gender, ethnicity and race. The Covid-19 pandemic has affected people from Black and Minority Ethnic communities more severely than other groups. The reasons for this are complex and influenced by multiple factors that must be analysed to determine how health services can respond more effectively to this serious inequality.

Effects of health inequalities

In England, people living in the poorest neighbourhoods will, on average, die 7 years earlier than people living in the richest neighbourhoods. In some areas this is even starker, with a 10 or 11 year difference. Another key factor is people in poorer areas will often experience more disability, so they will not only die sooner, but also spend more of their lives with a disability (Figure 22.1).

Health inequalities do not just affect health and social care; the repercussions for the economy are highly significant. It is estimated that inequality in illness in the UK accounts for productivity losses of £31–33 billion per year, lost taxes and higher welfare payments in the range of £20–32 billion per year, and additional NHS healthcare costs in excess of £5.5 billion per year. The cost of treating illnesses that result from inequalities in obesity alone are predicted to rise from £2 billion per year to nearly £5 billion per year by 2025.

The Marmot review gave six key recommendations for reducing health inequalities:

A – Give every child the best start in life.
B – Enable all children, young people and adults to maximise their capabilities and have control over their lives.
C – Create fair employment and good work for all.
D – Ensure healthy standard of living for all.
E – Create and develop healthy and sustainable places and communities.
F – Strengthen the role and impact of ill health prevention.

'Hard to reach' groups

Any individual can encounter health inequalities, but those who are homeless, endure mental illness, have a learning disability, are involved in offending or sex work, and those who have poor health literacy are often the ones who encounter the greatest inequalities in our society. Nurses may have limited impact on some of the causes of these inequalities, but can contribute greatly to their mitigation. A major opportunity is being able to engage with vulnerable groups. Often these individuals, families and groups are referred to as 'hard to reach', but the argument should rather be how we reach them (Figure 22.2).

Individuals may not present themselves readily to healthcare staff, but have networks of their own. Substance users rely on each other to obtain drugs, so this has been used by some services as a way to reach people through their peers. Homeless people use shelters and this presents an opportunity for outreach and health interventions. Offenders have to engage with staff in the criminal justice system, both in and out of prison.

To engage effectively, nurses should work closely with partner agencies who are involved with specific groups and, crucially, with the individuals themselves. Engaging someone who has a long-standing distrust and lack of confidence in health professionals is difficult, so any opportunity should be taken to bridge this divide. The chances of an individual returning for a follow-up appointment may be limited, so nurses should plan to use opportunistic encounters to the maximum effect. Taking these windows of opportunity can make a realistic and sustainable impact on that person's health.

23 Hygiene in the home, infection prevention and control

Susan Wynne, QN

Figure 23.1 Handwashing diagrams that can be shown to patients.

1 Apply 1 to 2 pumps of product to palms of dry hands.
2 Rub hands together, palm to palm.
3 Rub in between and around fingers.
4 Rub back of each hand with palm of other hand.
5 Rub fingertips of each hand in opposite palm.
6 Rub each thumb clasped in opposite hand.
7 Rub each wrist clasped in opposite hand.
8 Rub hands until product is dry. Do not use paper towels.

Figure 23.2 Transmission routes of micro-organisms.

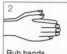

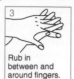

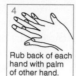

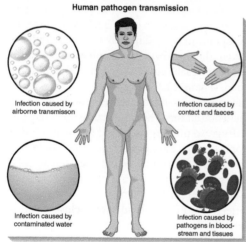

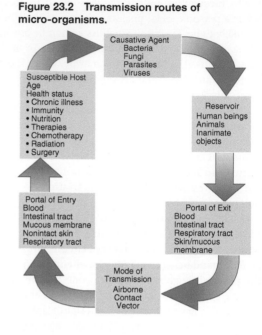

Causative Agent
Bacteria
Fungi
Parasites
Viruses
Reservoir
Human beings
Animals
Inanimate objects
Portal of Exit
Blood
Intestinal tract
Respiratory tract
Skin/mucous membrane
Mode of Transmission
Airborne
Contact
Vector
Portal of Entry
Blood
Intestinal tract
Mucous membrane
Nonintact skin
Respiratory tract
Susceptible Host
Age
Health status
• Chronic illness
• Immunity
• Nutrition
• Therapies
• Chemotherapy
• Radiation
• Surgery

Figure 23.3 Human pathogen transmission.

Human pathogen transmission
Infection caused by airborne transmisson
Infection caused by contact and faeces
Infection caused by contaminated water
Infection caused by pathogens in blood-stream and tissues

Figure 23.4 Hand hygiene at the point of care.

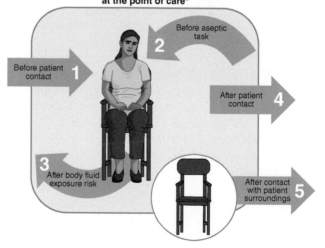

Your 5 moments for hand hygiene at the point of care*
1 Before patient contact
2 Before aseptic task
3 After body fluid exposure risk
4 After patient contact
5 After contact with patient surroundings

District Nursing at a Glance, First Edition. Edited by Matthew Bradby.

Infection prevention and control is an applied discipline associated with the prevention of nosocomial or healthcare-associated infection. Over the last decade, it has become a major political and patient safety concern, due to the level of mortality and morbidity related to MRSA bacteraemia and *Clostridium difficile* infection during inpatient hospital care. This has led to greater government-enforced controls and monitoring to improve patient outcomes. The impact of the Covid-19 pandemic has further illustrated the critical importance of effective hygiene in preventing infection.

Community nursing has advanced in tandem with the earlier discharge of patients from hospital, leading to developments in practice and new services. In the home, practitioners are faced with various challenges in minimising the risk of infection, including lack of control over environmental cleanliness, social deprivation, nutritional deficit, pets, pest infestation or poor living conditions. Despite this, intravenous therapy, renal dialysis, catheterisation, wound management, end-of-life care and a multitude of other interventions are now provided in the patient's own home.

The controls that have been instrumental in reducing infection rates in hospital are less practical within the community. When entering a patient's home, practitioners need to judge how suitable the environment will be for providing clinical care and must be able to undertake a risk assessment in order to manage potential problems. For instance, some patients may be colonised with MRSA, potentially placing them at risk of acquiring a bacteraemia, particularly if they have a venous access site or other invasive device. This risk assessment is based on the patient, environment, intervention and how many other people are engaged in the care of the patient.

Patient factors

To cause significant infection, bacterial microorganisms, viruses, fungi or parasites require a mode of transmission to a host. Age, physical condition, immune system, skin integrity and chemotherapy treatment are all important factors for assessing susceptibility to infection. Microorganisms will take advantage of poor host immunity, breaks in skin integrity such as a pressure or leg ulcer, or any other area that yields a mode of entry into the human host. This can be facilitated by direct or indirect contact (Figure 23.1).

Microorganisms can be passed from person to person by direct contact with body surfaces, such as touching, kissing, sexual contact or fluid from bodily lesions. Other direct modes of spread are by inhalation, ingestion, inoculation or transplacental (mother to infant) transmission. The risk of transmission of coronavirus in the home – airborne or on contaminated surfaces – should be carefully assessed in accordance with the latest public health guidelines.

Examples of direct transmission:

- *Inhalation*: breathing in *Legionella* bacterium via aerosols (small water droplets) direct from ventilation systems
- *Ingestion*: food-borne illnesses caused by bugs such as *Salmonella* or *Campylobacter*
- *Inoculation*: sharps injury potentially transmitting blood-borne viruses
- *Transplacental*: hepatitis B.

Transmission by indirect contact

Indirect infection can occur where disease agents are transmitted by a host to another on animate or inanimate objects, such as airborne particles, hands, medical devices, food, water or other vectors. Microorganisms are usually unable to travel within the air in isolation, but can be transmitted by particles, such as dust, water and respiratory secretions (Figure 23.2).

Large droplets from coughing, sneezing or talking can be expelled into the environment and inhaled by the patient. Smaller droplet nuclei can remain airborne for longer, potentially carrying organisms that can settle onto an open wound to cause infection. Keeping the patient's home care environment clean is therefore important for reducing the risk posed by the local bioburden (Figure 23.3).

To reduce the risk of wound infection, strict aseptic non-touch technique (ANTT) should be used to dress wounds, or when undertaking any other invasive procedure. Standard precautions should be applied for personal care and for body fluid spillage. Infections cause pain and discomfort for patients, potentially being responsible for months of rehabilitation or treatment. They can also be responsible for the demise of compromised patients who have succumbed to sepsis.

Equipment and fomites

Dust in the environment contains skin squames which are constantly shed from the skin surface. The dust can then settle on fomites within the environment, such as table tops, floors, bedding or medical equipment. Equipment that is well maintained, clean and dry does not support the growth of microorganisms. However, if equipment in frequent contact with a patient is contaminated with body fluids, there is an increased risk of microbial growth and risk of cross-infection. Simple damp dusting and using disinfectant after using the toilet or commode are advised, as well as handwashing before and after contact with the patient. The patient should also be offered handwashing cleansers if bed bound or assisted to wash hands regularly (Figure 23.4).

Medical devices such as hoists, commodes, walking frames and other care appliances need to be cleaned if visibly soiled with body fluids, and disinfection is required if commodes or toilets are soiled with faeces. Specialist beds should be inspected for integrity and any odours should be investigated. Smells may be due to the mattress if body fluids have permeated the integrity of the lining, increasing the risk of cross-infection in wounds.

Although practitioners are not responsible for cleaning in a patient's home, education of the family or patient is essential for reducing risk. Advice should be given to relatives or carers attending to the patient, such as social care workers, if they are providing care.

24 Substance and alcohol dependence

Alison Ward, QN

Box 24.1   Alcohol use disorders identification test (AUDIT). AUDIT is a comprehensive 10-question alcohol harm screening tool. It was developed by the World Health Organization and modified for use in the UK and has been used in a variety of health and social care settings.

Questions	Scoring system					Your score
	0	**1**	**2**	**3**	**4**	
How often do you have a drink containing alcohol?	Never	Monthly or less	2 to 4 times per month	2 to 3 times per week	4 times or more per week	
How many units of alcohol do you drink on a typical day when you are drinking?	0 to 2	3 to 4	5 to 6	7 to 9	10 or more	
How often have you had 6 or more units if female, or 8 or more if male, on a single occasion in the last year?	Never	Less than monthly	Monthly	Weekly	Daily or almost daily	
How often during the last year have you found that you were not able to stop drinking once you had started?	Never	Less than monthly	Monthly	Weekly	Daily or almost daily	
How often during the last year have you failed to do what was normally expected from you because of your drinking?	Never	Less than monthly	Monthly	Weekly	Daily or almost daily	
How often during the last year have you needed an alcoholic drink in the morning to get yourself going after a heavy drinking session?	Never	Less than monthly	Monthly	Weekly	Daily or almost daily	
How often during the last year have you had a feeling of guilt or remorse after drinking?	Never	Less than monthly	Monthly	Weekly	Daily or almost daily	
How often during the last year have you been unable to remember what happened the night before because you had been drinking?	Never	Less than monthly	Monthly	Weekly	Daily or almost daily	
Have you or somebody else been injured as a result of your drinking?	No		Yes, but not in the last year		Yes, during the last year	
Has a relative or friend, doctor or other health worker been concerned about your drinking or suggested that you cut down?	No		Yes, but not in the last year		Yes, during the last year	
Total AUDIT score						

Scoring:

- 0 to 7 indicates low risk
- 8 to 15 indicates increasing risk
- 16 to 19 indicates higher risk,
- 20 or more indicates possible dependence

Giving feedback and advice

- If the score is lower
- If the score is 8 or above, give <u>brief advice</u> to reduce risk for alcohol harm. If the score is 20 or above, consider referral to specialist alcohol harm assessment.

Alcohol unit reference

One unit of alcohol				

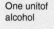 Half pint of "regular" beer, lager or cider   Half a small glass of wine   1 single measure of spirits   1 small glass of sherry   1 single measure of aperitifs

Drinks more than a single unit

 2 Pint of "regular" beer, lager or cider   **3** Pint of "strong" or "premium" beer, lager or cider   **1.5** Alcopop or a 275 ml bottle of regular lager   **2** 440 ml can of "regular" lager or cider   **4** 440 ml can of "super strength" lager   **3** 250 ml glass of wine (12%)    **9** 75 cl Bottle of wine (12%)

District Nursing at a Glance, First Edition. Edited by Matthew Bradby.
© 2022 John Wiley & Sons Ltd. Published 2022 by John Wiley & Sons Ltd.

Community nurses are in a prime position to identify health concerns in patients and families regarding drug and alcohol misuse, as part of a holistic assessment. Identifying substance misuse and harmful use of alcohol means these issues can then be integrated into care planning strategies involving health promotion and prevention of substance use. District nurses play an integral part in identifying safeguarding concerns relating to children in the home. They have a responsibility to alert the children's safeguarding board if there are any concerns that the parents' behaviour is causing harm – physically, socially or emotionally.

Substance misuse

Substance misuse refers to the harmful or hazardous use of psychoactive substances, including alcohol and illicit drugs. Psychoactive substances can lead to dependence syndrome – a cluster of behavioural, cognitive and physiological problems that occur after repeated use.

The most frequently reported misused drugs are cannabis, nitrous oxide, amphetamines, ecstasy and cocaine. Cannabis is the most commonly used drug in the UK. Cocaine, amphetamine and opioids present with the most significant health problems. A large proportion of individuals that misuse drugs are poly-drug users, not limiting their use to one particular drug. The likelihood of substance misuse is influenced by availability, peer pressure, social background and vulnerability. Obtaining substances can often lead to participating in criminal activity to fund the addiction. Novel psychoactive substances (NPS), artificially manufactured drugs, are presenting an increasing problem. Opioid misuse is often a long-term condition with periods of remission and relapse, and abstinence is not always achieved. Signs of misuse can present as irrational behaviours, dilated pupils, pink eyes, excessive eating, and boils on arms, legs, hands, groins and feet.

Common characteristics of individuals with substance use disorder may present as problems functioning in everyday life, causing individual psychological distress and a tendency to engage in dangerous behaviours. Individuals typically have increasing difficulty in recovering from the effects of substances, in reducing the amount used or being able to stop using them. This leads to an increased physical tolerance to the substance, with withdrawal symptoms occurring when the substance is metabolised and the effects wear off.

Pharmacological approaches are the primary treatment for opioid misuses, along with providing psychosocial interventions. For cannabis and stimulant misuse pharmacological treatments are not available, and psychosocial interventions are the only treatment. Treatment of dependence can be accessed via local authority/NHS specialist services to set up interventions and care plans to support and monitor the individual. Family or carer support may also be available via children's services, voluntary services or youth trusts, for access to alternative therapies, parent support and counselling.

Alcohol dependence

Alcohol is the most common drug involved in substance use disorder. Alcohol and its effects are a growing health concern as more people are drinking above the recommended daily safe limits. People often present at GP surgeries because of associated co-morbid effects of alcohol. Persons with an alcohol disorder typically develop a high tolerance for alcohol and will experience withdrawal symptoms if their access to it is suddenly stopped.

Alcohol intoxication can lead to immediate problems for the individual and others during excessive use. Alcohol dependence is linked to physical, mental and social problems, oesophageal varices, falls, hypertension, liver cirrhosis, diabetes, renal failure, seizures, toxicity, anxiety and dementia. Family relationships often break down leading to depression, aggression, loss of work and homelessness. There is also severe risk to the welfare of children whose parents have substance use disorders.

Care, management and prevention

Health professionals are in prime position to screen for consumption of excess alcohol. A questionnaire can be issued at wellbeing health checks and initial registration medicals. The 'gold standard' tool is the AUDIT-C for alcohol (the alcohol use disorders identification test) (Box 24.1). Questions are answered in a consultation, and if the individual scores 5 or more, this would lead to a full assessment. The score equates to the risk to the individual:

- 0–7   Lower risk
- 8–15   Increased risk – hazardous drinking = advice
- 16–19 Higher risk – harmful drinking = extensive intervention
- 20–40 Possible dependence

Recommended UK sensible drinking limits

- <14 units a week for men and women
- Two alcohol-free days a week advised
- Alcohol should be avoided in pregnancy due to the risk of fetal alcohol syndrome in the unborn child.

For a dependent drinker, reducing harm is the first priority. To stop consumption suddenly can cause adverse psychological effects, including tremors, anxiety and being unable to physically function. Therefore, a stepped approach to controlled drinking is required. Referrals can be made to Alcoholics Anonymous, specialist alcohol services locally such as NHS support services, and also family support for carers and children of dependent drinkers.

Education via schools, youth groups, health visitors, parenting groups, and GP surgeries can be given to supply appropriate information on the risks of alcohol on health and how to reduce harm. Education can help people recognise potential or current problems with their consumption levels. Encouraging positive changes and the opportunity to make changes with support may improve outcomes.

25 Safety in the home, including falls prevention

Helen Davies, QN

Box 25.1 Safety in the home (including falls prevention)

1 Ensure traffic areas both in and outdoors are clear and encourage repairs to be undertaken to any damaged areas to reduce risk of trips or falls.
2 Inspect and, if necessary, carry out repairs on any uneven surfaces or stairs, any change in height of the walkway should prompt further assessment and referral for consideration of handrails.
3 Consider using a non-slip material in the bath, shower and also under rugs. The patient's footwear should be well fitting, preferably with non-slip soles.
4 Loose rugs/mats, cords and cables under rugs or lying around can cause trips/falls: if it is not possible to remove them, consider securing them in each corner and include a non-slip material underneath to prevent slips and trips.
5 Patients with poor eyesight or cognitive impairment such as dementia may not be able to differentiate between differing heights of flooring. Using a contrasting colour at the top and bottom of the stairs or at the change in height level of the floor can help reduce falls.
6 Suggest regular vision checks. If the patient is housebound, check which opticians will do home visits and encourage the patient to wear glasses if needed.
7 Encourage use of proper lighting both in and outdoors around the home, with nightlights to assist with identification of a safe path to walk from bedroom to bathroom and kitchen.
8 A referral for handrails and other equipment in the bathroom to assist the patient with getting in and out of the bath/shower will improve safety and promote independence.
9 Caregivers should use any equipment provided to ensure safety, especially with transfers.
10 Consider referral to the physiotherapist and occupational therapist for assessment of need around equipment needed to improve the patient's gait and improve independence.
11 Falls prevention teams: Intermediate care, including rapid response teams, can provide this service, particularly where the patient is identified as high risk or has a history of falling. Intermediate care can also provide the patient with targeted therapy to improve function and promote confidence.
12 Encourage the patient to use any prescribed mobility equipment, especially where a balance or physical weakness may increase the risk of falling.
13 Use of telecare such as audio and/or video monitoring, falls alarms and bed and chair monitors can improve safety and ensure that a 'no-response' by the patient is quickly identified and help sent promptly. Patients can wear a neck pendent or bracelet which has a button they can press to summon help if they fall or become unwell. Bracelets can be activated automatically if the patient falls. This type of alarm is good for frequent falls or where the patient has an impairment where they are unable to recognise that they need help.
14 Information should be documented to aid any responder attending the patient in an emergency situation, so they have immediate access to emergency contact numbers and details of medical conditions. Documentation can be stored in a variety of ways. If, for example, it is in a plastic case in the fridge then a sticker should be put on the fridge door to indicate this.
15 General safety guidance on actions such as installation of carbon monoxide alarms, smoke alarms, key safe outside and general maintenance should be considered; approved companies can be sourced via local adult social care and, if available, a single point of access for patients and professionals.
16 Changing seasons can bring particular hazards, such as snow and ice outdoors. Access to snow clearing and application of salt to prevent falls may be provided by locally approved volunteer groups if the patient does not have family or neighbours who can help out.
17 Encourage the patient to keep warm in winter to avoid hypothermia, check they have enough food and access to fluids. In summer, they may need encouragement to increase fluid intake to avoid dehydration. Either extreme of being too hot or too cold can cause someone to fall.
18 Consider re-arranging the kitchen cupboards so that frequently used items are easier to reach. If necessary, encourage the patient to ask someone else to reach higher items and to use appropriate sturdy steps to avoid over-reaching or climbing onto work surfaces.
19 The patient should avoiding wearing loose clothing that could catch fire if too close to appliances such as cookers, fires or hot surfaces. Use of firefighting equipment such as fire blankets or extinguishers can be useful in the kitchen if the patient or caregiver knows how to use the items correctly.
20 Oven gloves should be used to remove hot items from the oven, hob or microwave to reduce risk of burns and scalds.
21 Medicine storage may involve a locked cupboard, box or carousel. Drugs such as insulin may need to be stored in the fridge. Consider who may be able to access medicines, including the patient, their caregiver, family or visitors with children. Use of child-proof containers may be needed alongside other measures such as a lock box.

Box 25.2 First aid for the home checklist.

- Use of telecare technology – pendent alarm/falls alert bracelet
- Smoke alarm and carbon monoxide alarm – 10-year battery or mains-operated
- Safe route of escape plan – in event of fire/flood/emergency evacuation
- Stay warm in winter/cool in summer
- Key safe to aid access to the home by carers/health professionals/emergency services
- Contact numbers for local gas and electricity
- Thermometers for rooms occupied
- Fireguard/fireblanket

The Royal Society for the Prevention of Accidents has a very useful website with more information regarding safety in the home and older people safety (https://www.rospa.com/home-safety/Advice/Older-People).

District Nursing at a Glance, First Edition. Edited by Matthew Bradby.
© 2022 John Wiley & Sons Ltd. Published 2022 by John Wiley & Sons Ltd.

As part of an holistic assessment, reviewing all aspects of the patient's condition and their environment is essential to ensuring they are able to function and live as safely and confidently as possible. Each person's home will be as different and individual as they are, however home safety is often overlooked when health professionals first visit the patient to assess/treat them for medical issues.

Staff health and safety should be of paramount concern when assessing suitability of the working environment – the patient's home. District nurses have been known to fall and injure themselves due to uneven paths, broken slabs, loose rugs and trailing cables and other hazards.

Each environment is usually risk assessed when first approached and often this information is passed on verbally or via electronic records. Specific information and potential dangers can be found as alerts in NHS and social care records. For example: 'Large dog – ring bell and family member will put dog in another room before entry'. As guests in the patient's home a partnership approach tends to work best, but as health professionals we have a duty of care to minimise the risks to the patient and ourselves.

Careful consideration is often needed when finding solutions to problems. For example, a patient having continuous oxygen therapy who had informed his consultant he no longer smoked, was found at home smoking whilst using his nasal cannula for his oxygen therapy. The patient had assumed he was allowed to smoke because he was not using a face mask. After re-educating the patient and building trust, a new plan was devised to minimise the risks involved; referring to pulmonary rehabilitation also helped him to reduce his smoking and reliance on oxygen. Another patient was often found by their carer falling asleep whilst smoking; the local fire service were asked to help with assessment and provided a fire blanket to minimise the risk of the patient harming themselves through fire.

Health professionals have an opportunity to educate and encourage the patient and their family/caregiver to address any health and safety risks, including the prevention of falls. The patient will decide whether or not to make any changes recommended by the health professional and this should always be documented in the care records. Where a patient lacks mental capacity, this should also be documented and any best interest decisions recorded with the agreed action plan to minimise risks.

Liaison with everyone involved in the care and welfare of the patient is needed. The lead worker could be a district nurse, or it may be another professional such as a social worker, community matron, mental health worker, learning disability nurse or case manager. Safety of vulnerable adults can also include the adult safeguarding team making specific recommendations to ensure the patient's best interest is being upheld.

There are four main areas to be considered when trying to lower your patient's falls risk: ensuring they have access to regular vision checks, improving balance and strength through exercise, making the home environment safer, and having regular reviews of medication.

Eyesight problems through wearing the wrong glasses, glaucoma or cataracts contribute to an increased risk of falling. Where a patient is housebound, check locally for opticians who can perform a home visit or help the patient to access services by referring them for appropriate transport solutions. Often third-party organisations such as the British Red Cross can help with this.

As the health professional, you can recommend appropriate exercises for the patient, refer them for occupational and/or physiotherapy, or refer them to intermediate care. Encourage participation in local groups such as tai chi, or chair-based exercise where appropriate. Any exercise which increases strength and improves balance will reduce the risk of falling; it will also make the patient feel better and more confident to move about.

Risks within the home can account for almost 50% of all falls and making changes at home can help to decrease the risk of falling significantly. Many people do not realise that as you get older, you need brighter lights to see properly, especially in darker corridors and on the stairs. Encourage the patient to wear shoes indoors rather than slippers or bare feet, to reduce the possibility of trips and slips leading to falls.

Conduct regular reviews of medication to identify risks associated with polypharmacy, dosage changes needed and other interactions.

General safety and falls prevention are interlinked and generally there are simple practical rules to be followed; for example, do not overload an electrical socket or adapters, use a cordless phone to avoid trailing flexes, remove magazines lying in the path walked by the patient, and place a walking frame within reach of the sitting patient (Box 25.1).

Frailty and poor health leading to accidents in older people account for a significant proportion of attendances to accident and emergency departments. A simple urinary tract infection in an older person can quickly become a significant risk, causing confusion and loss of balance leading to a fall, resulting in fractured bones requiring surgery or periods in hospital (Box 25.2). Older people have a slower recovery time and may need intensive support to help them regain their independence, demonstrating the importance that falls prevention initiatives play in promoting home safety and welfare.

Effective discharge planning

Lena O'Reilly, QN

Table 26.1 Distinguishing between simple and complex health and social care needs.

Simple ongoing care needs do not require complex planning and delivery. For example:	Complex ongoing care needs require detailed assessment planning and delivery by a multiprofessional team and with multi-agency working. The indicators for use could be:
• The patient does not require or want any social care services in discharge	• Use of the Barthel Activities of Daily Living Index assessment tool, which would show a high dependency care was needed
• The patient requires straightforward community nurse services on discharge, such as dressings or suture removal	• The patient was receiving community or social care services prior to hospital admission
• The patient does not require or want any social care services in discharge	• If there is a need for assessment for the use of nursing equipment, syringe drivers or pressure-relieving mattresses, ongoing rehabilitation at home or if the home environment is unsafe.
• The patient is independent or has a carer	

Further comprehensive lists can be obtained from 'Ready to go?' document (Department of Health, 2010).

Figure 26.1   The individual being cared for may receive support from numerous professionals on discharge from hospital, including the District Nursing service.

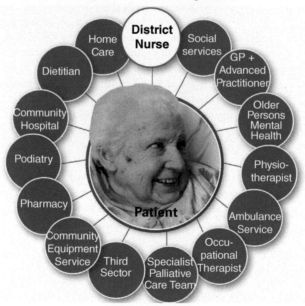

Patient empowerment is embedded in nursing philosophy, so the approach to discharge planning should also be patient-centred. Good communication is essential and plays a pivotal role in forming productive relationships between the nurse, patient, carers and family.

Planned care

Currently, collaborative working between disciplines, agencies and departments to enable planned care to progress to discharge requires specific actions to take place, including decisions on the process and the timings of the transfer or discharge.

The Department of Health and Social Care (formerly Department of Health) identified 10 steps in the transfer/discharge process, as described in the document 'Ready to go?' (Department of Health, 2010). This clearly states the first step should be to start planning discharge before or on admission. This is crucial to the identification of any issues that may make the discharge difficult, so that action can be taken to ensure good planned care. On admission, all medication should be reviewed, a medicines care plan put into place and training in treatment concordance given.

Developing a clinical management plan, setting out the goals for the patient, identifying barriers and methods of overcoming these, test therapies and other interventions, are ideally completed within the first 24 hours of admission. Assessment and good coordination by the multidisciplinary team is essential to ensure that everyone understands their role and responsibilities. Although early proactive care planning is essential, it is important not to prejudge the eventual outcomes for the patient before their full potential is achieved. Rehabilitation potential should always be explored and acted upon before any life-changing decisions are made (Figure 26.1).

Effective coordination of the discharge or transfer process continues with effective leadership and handover responsibility at ward level. This will have a significant impact on the quality and speed of the patient's journey. It is vital for one person to be accountable for leading the care planning process each day, with all the relevant information available to them. The ward handover will identify the future care coordinator. Up-to-date documentation is indispensable, with a central file for all team members to contribute information to the plan. Many wards now use the system of boards to improve the communication between staff.

Predicted length of stay can be estimated according to various factors. One is the way ward performance is measured, as the estimated date for discharge is often based on the time required for test and interventions to be completed, the integrated care pathway followed, and the time it is likely to take for the patient to be clinically stable and fit for discharge. Simple discharges should be within 24 hours and non-urgent tests can be undertaken as an outpatient. For complex cases, it can be more difficult to anticipate the length of stay, so multidisciplinary assessment and planning will be required.

Patient-centred care

Once the initial assessment has been completed, staff need to identify whether the patient has simple or complex discharge/transfer needs, involving the patient and carer (Table 26.1). This is managed primarily by the multidisciplinary team, which should identify these complexities early in the patient's journey.

Using terminology that is familiar to the patient is important to ensure that the right questions are asked, so that their lifestyle is clearly established prior to admission, and to understand the role of the carer, as their views may differ from those of the patient. Bear in mind that the patient is the expert on how they feel and how they would like to be involved in decision-making. Patients and carers should feel empowered to manage their care, rehabilitation and transfer/discharge.

Patients are usually given an expected date of discharge or transfer within 24–48 hours of admission; this should be discussed with them and their family. Most patients and families want to know how long the inpatient stay is likely to be, what sort of treatment they are to receive and when they are likely to be discharged. Discharge planning with the patient should focus on their own goals and plans for their own discharge or transfer.

It is acceptable for a person to move from an acute ward to an interim placement until a permanent choice becomes available. Occasionally, someone who is approaching the end of their life may be admitted inappropriately. In such cases, where they do not wish to die in hospital, care plans should be put into place to enable then to be discharged quickly and safely so they can die with dignity in the place of their choice.

It is important to identify likely problems in a patient's care pathway, for example by a daily review of the clinical management plan with the patient, taking necessary actions and updating the discharge date. The majority of common conditions have integrated care pathways, and these should be used where available to enable practitioners to anticipate and plan. Always involve the patient and their family and carers.

Planning discharges and transfers should deliver continuity of care for all patients. This is regardless of the day of the week that the patient is admitted, allowing for adjustments to be put into place and compensating for a reduced length of stay in some cases. A discharge checklist, completed 24–48 hours prior to discharge or transfer, will enable good effective working between the patient and their family and the members of the ward core multidisciplinary team, including community providers.

27 Encouraging patient concordance

Gina Riley, QN

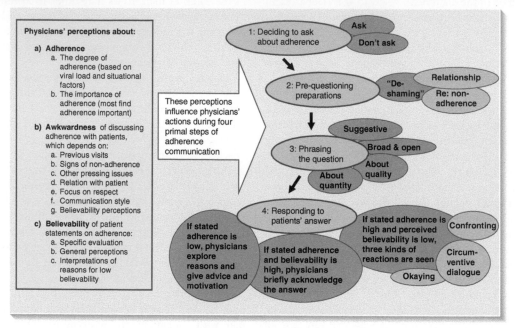

Figure 27.1   Model of physicians' adherence communication (expanded version). Physicians go through four steps when communicating with patients about adherence. The way physicians act in these is markedly influenced by three aspects of their perceptions. Each of the four steps has its subcategories, and each of the three perceptions has its main determinants. Source: Barfod, T.S., Hecht, F.M., Rubow, C. and Gerstoft, J. (2006). Physicians' communication with patients about adherence to HIV medication in San Francisco and Copenhagen: a qualitative study using Grounded Theory. *BMC Health Services Research* 6(1): 154. Licensed under CC BY 2.0.

Figure 27.2   Discussing a care plan with a patient one-to-one is key to effective communication and adherence. Explaining the risks and benefits of the treatment or care plan to your patient is crucial to allow them to to be concordant by making an informed choice in negotiating treatment or care options. Negotiating skills are required to enable discussions to take place between you and your patient about the care that they wish to have to facilitate patient concordance and compliance.

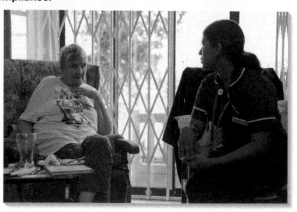

Box 27.1   Five dimension of adherence according to the World Health Organization (2003).

- Social and economic factors
- Health system/healthcare team-related factors
- Therapy-related factors
- Condition-related factors
- Patient-related factors

Patient concordance is a strategy that forms part of a treatment plan that seeks to promote patient wellbeing and prevent harm. The term concordance (or adherence) is used where a patient and the health professional discuss treatment options and agree a treatment or care plan together; however non-concordance is frequently a problem. If concordance relies on forming effective relationships, factors that could undermine this would be distrust, poor communication, poor information sharing or failure to agree a plan.

There are many reasons and factors that contribute to concordance and compliance with health education, health promotion, treatments and advice. The World Health Organization has identified five main dimensions of adherence (Box 27.1).

The term non-concordance is often used where patients refuse to take some or all of their medication as prescribed, but the term non-adherence will also be encountered. Medication non-adherence is a growing concern because of mounting evidence that it is prevalent and associated with adverse outcomes.

In the community, district nurses will work with many patients who are non-concordant. Patients can be non-concordant with treatment for many reasons. Side effects – actual and/or perceived – are a common reason as to why a patient stops taking their medication. If a patient believes that their medication is giving them particular symptoms, this may be why they stop taking it. Not knowing what their medication is actually for can be another reason why patients may not take it. Within community nursing, patient non-concordance is much more likely to occur than when nursing a patient in hospital, as the patient is not monitored on a 24-hour basis. Often the problem occurs when there is a breakdown in communication and if the patient feels that they have valid reasons for not taking the advice of the district nurse. In some cases, the negotiation process around treatment options and care plans may not be carried out as well as it should be for the patient to be truly concordant (Figures 27.1 and 27.2).

In the community, these issues can be difficult to overcome, as the district nurse is a guest in the patient's home and has a duty to respect the patient's choices, providing there is no reason to doubt the patient's mental capacity to make decisions for themselves. Within district nursing there are many situations where the patient may choose not to take advice or declines the opportunity to discuss and agree the treatment options, which may result in harm. Three of the most common areas of non-concordance are pressure area care, leg ulcer management and pain management, which will be discussed in more depth.

Patients who are assessed as being at risk of developing pressure ulcers may decline the provision of pressure-relieving equipment such as mattresses and cushions. Some patients may accept the use of a mattress but insist on using inappropriate bedding such as blankets on the mattress or incontinence sheets which will conversely affect the pressure-relieving properties of the mattress. A non-concordant patient may also discuss and agree to use a cushion but then be frequently found to be not sitting on the cushion when the district nurse visits. It is extremely important that the patient is given both written and verbal information about the risks of developing pressure ulcers and how they can be prevented. Often it is this discussion and information giving that assists the patient in complying with the advice, or discussing and agreeing the plan of care that is being recommended.

Similarly, some patients who require compression therapy for venous leg ulcers are unable to tolerate this treatment and are therefore non-concordant with the treatment recommended to heal the leg ulcers. Some patients will refuse this treatment without trying it and others will commence the therapy but then take the compression bandages off as they are unable to tolerate the discomfort of wearing them. One of the reasons why some patients do not tolerate the compression therapy is because they feel that the bandages are too tight and cause pain. Explaining why the compression bandages are needed and how they work to heal the leg ulcers may help the patient to understand the benefit of following the treatment. Other treatment options may be discussed with the patient, as there are different types of bandaging systems available and agreement may be negotiated if the patient is given a choice to trial different bandages.

Some patients, particularly those who are suffering from pain, may take their analgesia, but not as regularly as they should and therefore still experience pain. In some cases patients may believe that the medication is not working because they are still experiencing pain and then stop taking the analgesia altogether. It is very important that the patient receives both verbal and written information about what the medication is for, how often they need to take it and how many tablets they need to take. If a particular medication is not suitable, there may be other non-medicinal pain relief options available that could be discussed with the patient. It is essential for patients to have an informed choice before a particular treatment plan is agreed.

If the patient is involved in the decision-making process and feels that their opinions, possible anxieties or previous experiences have been listened to, concordance is more likely to result. Similarly, if patients are given information and the opportunity to ask questions about other treatment options that are available, they are more likely to be concordant with the advice being given.

28 Community health equipment services

Candice Pellett, QN

Figure 28.1   A clinical bed provided for use in a person's home.

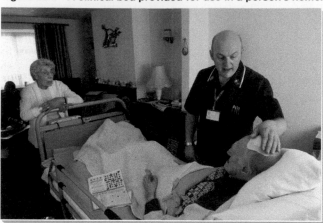

Figure 28.2   Assisting a person with mobility issues with eating and drinking.

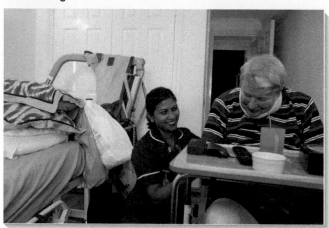

Figure 28.3   Supporting an elderly woman in the use of specialist equipment at home. Source: John Hopkins/Alamy.

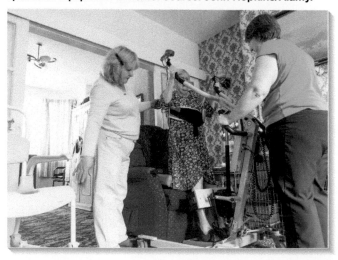

District Nursing at a Glance, First Edition. Edited by Matthew Bradby.
© 2022 John Wiley & Sons Ltd. Published 2022 by John Wiley & Sons Ltd.

Community health equipment services provide health and social care equipment to meet the needs of residents, from simple aids for daily living to more complex pieces of equipment to enable people to stay in their home environment. Most regions have a community or joint equipment store, which is funded by the local authority and the NHS.

Supply of equipment

Equipment is available, subject to the assessed need of the patient, to assist in:

- Hospital admission avoidance
- Discharge from hospital
- Nursing at home
- Preventing further deterioration
- Maintaining independence at home
- Enabling the statutory agencies to meet appropriate regulations for their staff, i.e. health and safety.

Simple aids can help support a person to maintain their independence with daily living. This may be an item such as a bath board to help a person get in and out of the bath or a raised toilet seat to help someone get on and off the toilet safely. Simple aids can assist people with bathing, meal preparation and eating, dressing and mobility. Complex aids are usually supplied by health and/or local authority to enable a person to remain in their home environment. Examples of complex aids include hoists, specialist beds, pressure mattress and bath lifts. These items often have complex or electrical parts and will require planned maintenance to keep them in safe working order (Figure 28.1).

Prescribing

Requests for equipment provision are usually made following an assessment from the professional involved in the patient's care. The prescriber must consider the needs of the patient as part of the care planning process and, where possible, the patient and their carer/family should be fully involved in how their needs are met and be informed about how to use the equipment safely.

It is imperative that assessment for, and prescribing of, equipment should only be made by a staff member who is qualified to do so, has attended relevant training, and has the skills and knowledge in this area of care. All assessments undertaken, including risk assessments, must be recorded using the appropriate documentation in line with the employer's policies (Figure 28.2). These must be updated following reassessment at a minimum of six months, or more frequently should the situation change. Some items of equipment must be prescribed with caution, for example, bed rails (also known as cot sides). This requires a full risk assessment to enable the prescriber to be certain that the bed rails are high enough to take into account any increased mattress thickness or additional overlay, to prevent the patient rolling over the top and to ensure that any gaps between rails, mattress, headboard and footboard do not present a serious risk of entrapment. Risk assessments should be undertaken before use and reviewed and recorded after each significant change in the patient's condition and regularly during the period of use.

Delivery of equipment

Most items of equipment are delivered between 2 and 5 days from prescription, although some non-stock items will take longer. Same-day delivery usually incurs an additional charge, but this may be necessary when a patient is at the end of life and deterioration is unexpectedly rapid, and to prevent admission or to aid hospital discharge when a patient is at end of life and wishes to be nursed and to die at home. Another example of the need for same-day delivery is for patients with deteriorating pressure ulcers where no pressure-relieving equipment is in place (perhaps resulting from a first assessment visit by the district nurse) or where the equipment requires upgrading urgently to prevent further breakdown of skin integrity.

Equipment for moving and handling

There are many items of equipment available to assist the patient with their dependency requirements. These include:

- Suitable walking aids
- Handrails
- Support poles/rails
- Wheelchairs
- Electric profiling beds for immobile/dependent patients
- Transfer boards and slide sheets
- Selection of hoists, standing aids, bath hoists, bariatric hoists
- Slings of different sizes and types to meet patients' needs.

It is paramount that safe working procedures are used whilst hoisting a patient, otherwise a serious incident may occur if the wrong type of hoist or sling is used, or if the incorrect size is used, as this may result in a patient falling or slipping through the sling.

Equipment should only be ordered following a holistic assessment of needs to enhance daily living and must be used in conjunction with a care plan and the manufacturer's instructions for use (Figure 28.3).

The district nursing team is well placed to recognise the signs if the patient is struggling to cope in their home and they can also refer to the community physiotherapy and occupational therapy services who provide care for patients at home by providing assessment, diagnosis, treatment and provision of equipment for patients with complex needs that are best met within their home environment.

Loss of independence has huge implications for the patient and their family/carer. Supporting the patient with appropriate equipment can facilitate an appropriate environment for the patient to remain safely in their own home.

29 The use of new technology to assist daily living in the home

Hilary Thompson, QN

Table 29.1 The benefits and challenges of using technology in the home.

Benefits	Challenges
• Takes into account individuals' needs and preferences and as such is person centred • Empowers people to have a better understanding of their condition, take ownership of their health and thus facilitates self-management and independence • Provides early detection of complications so intervention can be timely to prevent deterioration of conditions and harm • Supports informal family carers to feel reassured and less anxious as they know the person is being monitored • Supports patient care and contributes to a positive patient experience • Reduces the time spent travelling by healthcare practitioners visiting patients who are house bound	• Patients require a contact person (family carer, friend, neighbour) to accept responsibility as a 'contact person' • Technology is not always available to district nurses in the form of computers, nor are all district nurses fully competent in the use of information technology • District nurses require training to understand and use assistive technology and protected time and resources to respond to work generated by telehealth care • There needs to be a clear understanding of processes and protocols as to how patient data and information will be shared and acted upon • This requires effective communication and good integrated working with health and social care colleagues over the 24-hour period

Figure 29.1   The internet allows for a permanent interface between remote devices and their human users. Source: FS Productions/Tetra images/Getty Images.

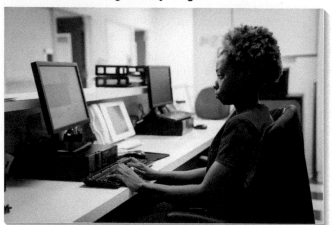

Understanding the health and social care landscape

The shift in focus of care from the hospital setting to the community has been driven by a number of factors. Demographic influences, namely a growth in the older population and a rise in the number of those people living with one or more long-term condition are important considerations which have underpinned the reshaping of services in the community.

Not only are these services aimed at addressing a person's existing health and social care needs, but they incorporate systems to facilitate the identification of potential health risks, thus providing the opportunity for interventions at an early stage to prevent complications and possible hospital admissions. The challenge of developing effective alternative community services for people living in their own homes takes into account the availability of new technological and digital solutions to support an individual's needs and preferences, as well as those of their families and informal carers (Figure 29.1).

Disease-specific specialist nurses, such as those caring for people living with dementia, stroke, diabetes, heart failure, epilepsy and chronic obstructive pulmonary disease, have embraced telehealth and telecare as a much valued and integral part of the care process.

Despite the benefits of telehealth and telecare for both the patient and clinician, new mobile technologies do not replace face-to-face physical contact but they do complement it (Table 29.1).

Nevertheless, many district nurses have not yet incorporated this within their practice. The pace of change has accelerated, however, with the impact of the Covid-19 pandemic, which has given new impetus to the use of remote monitoring technology, for example for people recovering at home after a hospital admission for Covid-19. The Queen's Nursing Institute website contains a number of case studies of new uses of remote technology in direct response to the pressures of the pandemic.

Associated definitions and terminology

- *Remote* refers to the place where the person lives (i.e. their own home).
- *eHealth* refers to all clinical records, data, information and care delivery that use any form of information and communication technology (ICT).
- *Connected health* encompasses health programmes in remote care.
- *Telehealth* records clinical observations remotely. Telehealth is the consistent and accurate monitoring of a patient's vital signs and symptoms via easy to use technology in their own home. The clinician (community nurse) is able to monitor the patient's clinical observations from her place of work. Technical triage personnel (at the support centre) verify the results and alert a clinician if the data are outside the parameters set for that individual patient (for patients who are triaged only).
- *Triage* refers to a support team who receive, interpret and prioritise patient data and communicate this to healthcare professionals
- *Track and trend* refers to the process whereby the clinician monitors a person's clinical observations and follows the established trend.
- *Telecare* provides remote systems/sensors for independent living. It helps to manage risk and supports people to live safely by the means of unobtrusive wireless sensors placed around the home which detect possible problems such as smoke, gas, flood or a person falling. On detecting any of the above, sensors automatically raise a local, audible alarm, as well as alerting a nominated carer, key holder, or the monitoring centre, as appropriate.

'Nursing in the digital age: using technology to support patients in the home' is a major report published by the Queen's Nursing Institute (QNI) in 2018. It seeks to determine how far new healthcare information technology has changed in recent years and how skills and attitudes within community services have adapted. The QNI's report identified that:

- there were at least 67 differently named IT systems in use in community healthcare;
- 74% of community nurses find IT systems a more reliable way of working, compared to paper;
- 29% of community nurses are still working largely with paper-based systems;
- 41% of NHS trusts do not use telehealth systems;
- 28% of services are utilising a text messaging facility to remind patients of their appointments.

Since the publication of that report, the Department of Health and Social Care has launched a new organisation, 'NHSX', which will help deliver new digital tools that can be used by all health professionals and support the delivery of person-centred care for patients, families and communities. Free webinars and other online training are now increasingly accessible and are often promoted in relevant social media.

30 Use of mobile technology to support practice

Margo Grady, QN

Figure 30.1   Community nurses are using mobile technology to create time to care.

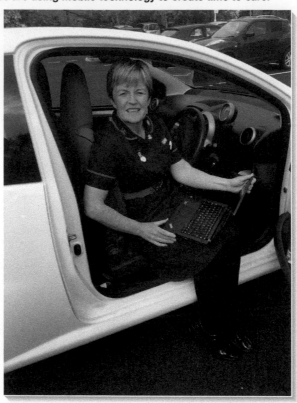

Figure 30.2   An example of a web-based work scheduling tool used in District Nursing, illustrating base and mobile user interfaces.

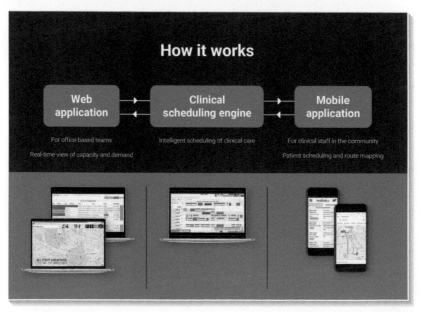

District Nursing at a Glance, First Edition. Edited by Matthew Bradby.
© 2022 John Wiley & Sons Ltd. Published 2022 by John Wiley & Sons Ltd.

District nursing is currently experiencing a transformation of digital care and integrated electronic healthcare records. Programmes are in use that will be able to schedule visits by time and location, thus saving time and money and freeing up capacity to make services more responsive. As well as ensuring no patient need is missed, these systems also improve staff safety and reduce hazards inherent in lone working.

In district nursing we need to optimise technology to support remote working. We work at the interface between primary and secondary care, which both strive to be paperless, but in many cases district nursing services continue to be reliant on paper. In recent years, spending on information technology in healthcare has increased enormously, which represents a huge cultural shift to maximise mobile working. This should increase time available for direct patient care.

Improving efficiency and creating capacity

Mobile technology can improve efficiency by allowing real-time recording of information directly to the patient's electronic record. Trials have shown that service capacity may increase dramatically simply because district nurses do not have to go to their base every morning to collect paper case notes. Less travel not only frees time but also saves significant amounts of money in mileage claims (Figure 30.1).

Nurses who have more clinical information are able to deliver higher quality care, reduce risk, demonstrate improved decision-making and are more likely to be able to keep patients out of hospital. The district nurse has the opportunity to plan, implement and evaluate care – and upload accurate contemporary records with less duplication of work.

Mobile working devices are portable and should be easy to use in the patient's home, with different teams using laptops or smartphones to gain remote access. The device will usually self-select the best connectivity, so the nurse will simply need to switch it on.

Staff training is key to the successful use of technology, as although nurses will have varied IT skills, additional training may be needed to use mobile devices to their full capability. If a district nurse moves area, where different systems are in use, full training should be given; systems everywhere will continue to develop and training must be ongoing in order to keep pace with improvements (Figure 30.2).

Patients as partners

The evidence is that more patients are being seen at home since the introduction of mobile working and these patients express satisfaction with the service delivered by nurses, not least because they do not have to attend further appointments to receive test results and other information that nurses can now share with them at home.

Supported self-management by patients is a key part of the NHS Long Term Plan and has become even more significant due to the impact of the Covid-19 pandemic.

There are numerous firms now facilitating telehealth for patients and offering monitoring of vital signs from the patient's home. This technology supports patients by recording their blood pressure, temperature, pulse and oxygen saturation and delivers the capability to upload these by internet or telephone. Structures can be put in place to contact the patient's lead clinician to report on any abnormalities in vital signs and alert to any changes. The nurse can then help facilitate early treatment of symptoms to prevent deterioration of the patient's condition and hospital admission.

Patients can be supported to manage their own condition via smartphone applications and this may ultimately result in less face-to-face contact. In addition, technology is now available for patients to perform certain blood tests on hand-held devices and text the results to a pathology laboratory. By return, the laboratory will advise on medication doses needed. This eliminates the need for blood tests previously performed by a nurse on a home visit. Programmes are constantly evolving and it is anticipated that there will be more smartphone applications to support patients in managing different long-term conditions.

Evolving solutions

Poor data connectivity can be a downside of the new mobile technology. This is not a problem that can be resolved easily, but district nurses familiar with their neighbourhood will be aware of areas where this is a problem and can plan ahead for this eventuality. This may entail inputting data when they arrive at an area with better connectivity. Already solutions to this problem are being developed, such as a programme to store information and forward it when connectivity is re-established. As mobile technology develops, we would expect this problem to resolve as it is regarded as a priority by system developers. The anticipated problem with patients accepting electronic patient records in their homes has been overstated and in fact patient satisfaction is high, once they become used to the new systems.

Time to care

Essentially, using mobile technology will focus on reducing the burden of paperwork and releasing time to care. As nurses we need to see technology used in mobile working as a tool and use the time it makes available to practise the art and science of nursing. This is not an end in itself but a route to improving the care we deliver, increasing capacity to give high-quality care to patients in their homes. Community nurses need to be ready to embrace the information revolution.

31 Patient care in nursing homes

Linda Thornley, QN, Charlotte Hudd, QN, and Anne Bennett, QN

Figure 31.1 Resident and nurse in a care home setting.

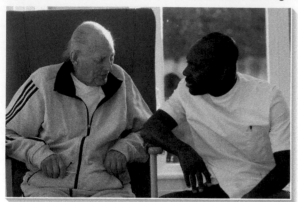

Figure 31.2 Residents and nurse in a care home setting.

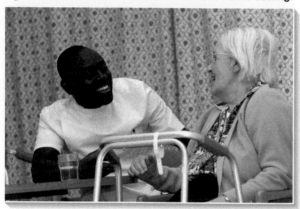

Table 31.1 Care Quality Commission: Key Lines of Enquiry.

Safe	• Are people safe? • Are people protected from abuse and harm?
Caring	• Do staff involve and treat people with compassion, kindness, dignity and respect?
Responsive	• Are services organised so that they meet people's needs?
Effective	• Does care, treatment and support achieve good outcomes? • Does it promote a good quality of life? • Is it based on best available evidence?
Well-led	• Do leadership, management and governance of the organisation assure the delivery of high-quality, person-centred care, support learning and innovation, and promote an open and fair culture?

Table 31.2 Care Quality Commission: Care home regulation.

Regulation 1	Citation and commencement
Regulation 2	Interpretation
Regulation 3	Prescribed activities
Regulation 4	Requirements where the service provider is an individual or partnership
Regulation 5	Fit and proper persons
Regulation 6	Requirement where the service provider is a body other than a partnership
Regulation 7	Requirements relating to registered managers
Regulation 8	General
Regulation 9	Person-centred care
Regulation 10	Dignity and respect
Regulation 11	Need for consent
Regulation 12	Safe care and treatment
Regulation 13	Safeguarding service users from abuse and improper treatment
Regulation 14	Meeting nutritional and hydration needs
Regulation 15	Premises and equipment
Regulation 16	Complaints
Regulation 17	Good governance
Regulation 18	Staffing
Regulation 19	Fit and proper persons employed
Regulation 20	Duty of candour
Regulation 20A	Requirement as to display of performance assessments
Regulation 21	Guidance and code
Regulation 22	Offences
Regulation 23	Offences – penalties
Regulation 24	Penalty notices
Regulation 25	Revocations
Regulation 26	Transitional and transitory provision
Regulation 27	Review

Care Quality Commission https://www.cqc.org.uk/

District Nursing at a Glance, First Edition. Edited by Matthew Bradby.
© 2022 John Wiley & Sons Ltd. Published 2022 by John Wiley & Sons Ltd.

Nursing homes are communities within a community. Nursing home communities commonly care for frail older people living with long-term conditions and most nursing homes are a permanent place of residency. However, some nursing home places may be used for patients on their journey from hospital back to their own home. Care homes differ from nursing homes in that they do not usually have full-time nursing staff (Figure 31.1).

Nursing in this setting is needed is for residents with life-limiting illness, multiple co-morbidities and complex mental health needs. These home communities may also be for ex-offenders and for children and for adults of all ages with complex mental and physical needs or learning disabilities. Nursing interventions in this setting could include:

- Administration of medication by injection
- Dressing of an open or closed wound
- Artificial feeding
- Basic nursing care of the type normally given to people who are confined to bed
- Intensive rehabilitation following surgery or disease
- Management of complex prostheses or appliances.

Registered nurses working in nursing homes are true autonomous practitioners. They need to be well-rounded, skilled, knowledgeable and effective. These skills are imperative to deliver good care. The nurse will most often be the only trained person on duty and will have to make complex decisions with just one chance to get it right. Care home nurses often have management responsibilities for staff at all levels of experience. District nurses may be called upon to visit a care home if a resident experiences an exacerbation of a long-term condition, or to provide additional staff training.

Demographics and regulation

The population of the UK is ageing: the number of people in the UK over 65 has increased by 21% over the past decade and the number of those over 85 has risen by 31% since 2005. This trend is predicted to grow. Hospitals are most suitable for short episodes of care and are not designed to provide ongoing care for people once their illness or injury has been treated and their condition stabilised. People requiring continuing care are better cared for in a purpose-designed environment (Figure 31.2). Residents often live with multiple co-morbidities, exacerbated by communication barriers as many in the care environment are living with dementia. This is where nursing homes are essential and it is especially true when palliative care is required.

Community care homes are regulated by the Care Quality Commission (CQC). The CQC ensures that all care is person-centred and that residents are true partners in decisions about their health and care, and that the home is safe, effective, caring, responsive and well-led. Inspectors use a set of standard Key Lines of Enquiry (KLOEs) which are linked to five key questions: Is your service safe, caring, responsive, effective and well-led? (Tables 31.1 and 31.2). These lead to a set of mandatory KLOEs that address the key priorities of every service.

Complex care: pain and dementia

When dementia causes behavioural and psychological symptoms, this may bring major trauma and distress to the individual concerned, their families and those who care for them. To enable good, safe, person-centred care, skills, knowledge, experience and expertise are required.

Assessment skills, understanding and being able to interpret what one sees, and the ability to anticipate need, are key. Disruptive vocalisation, physical and verbal aggression, and agitation are often key features which are the most challenging to manage. Staff have to be able to recognise potential triggers and unmet needs. These often include the individual being too hot, too cold, tired, hungry or thirsty. Underlying long-term conditions, co-morbidities, infection, pain and noise, the environment and overcrowding also need to be considered.

Pain in advanced dementia is one of the most common symptoms that people experience and is often poorly recognised. Pain then manifests in challenging behaviours. Nurses working in care homes are a valuable resource because they often know their residents well and can identify when pain is the root cause. It is good practice to use a pain assessment tool such as the Disability Distress Assessment Tool (DIsDAT). The first intervention will often be a simple analgesia, such as paracetamol. The key is to administer regularly and on time. Ensure that pain relief is part of the care-planning process, with thorough assessment and regular evaluation.

Hospice at home

The nurse is in a prime position to identify and respond to patients nearing the end of life. The role involves working as part of a supportive team to provide 24-hour care, monitor health conditions, administer medication, use medical devices, and advise patients and their families on current prognosis. The nursing home nurse is in an ideal position to develop trusting, flexible and sustainable relationships with the family, as often the patient will reside in the home for a period of months or years.

The QNI operates a Care Home Nurses Network with online events and learning materials. For more information visit: https://www.qni.org.uk/nursing-in-the-community/care-home-nurses-network/

32 Person-centred dementia care

Mo Boersma, QN

Figure 32.1 Key contributors to effective person-centred dementia care in the community.

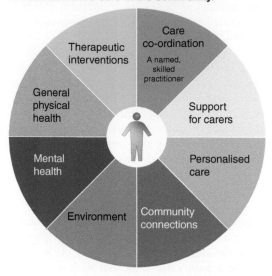

Figure 32.2 Some key elements in person-centred care for individuals.

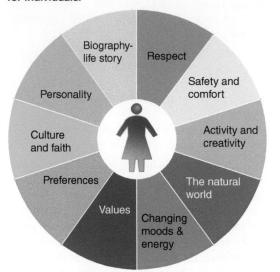

Table 32.1 Cognitive impacts and behavioural effects of Dementia.

Cognitive Impairment	Behavioural Manifestation	Functional Limitations
Memory	Personality, behavioural and mood changes	Self-care
Confusion	Apathy	Activities of daily living
Concentration	Anger	Balance and gait
Disorientation	Anxiety	Motor skills
Language	Sleep disturbance	Visuo-spatial diffculties
Learning capacity	Delusions	
Judgement	Hallucinations	
Comprehension	Physical aggression	
Calculation	Depression	
Time perception	Disinhibited social behaviour	

District Nursing at a Glance, First Edition. Edited by Matthew Bradby.
© 2022 John Wiley & Sons Ltd. Published 2022 by John Wiley & Sons Ltd.

Dementia

Dementia is an umbrella term for a range of progressive conditions that affect the brain by damaging the neurons and preventing messages being relayed effectively within the brain. Dementia UK describes dementia as a collection of symptoms including a decline in memory, reasoning and communication. In conjunction with cognitive failure there is a parallel decline in function and skills required to carry out routine daily activities. There are over 200 subtypes of dementia, but the five most common are: Alzheimer's disease, vascular dementia, dementia with Lewy bodies, fronto-temporal dementia and mixed dementia. Dementia can be diagnosed at any age but is most common in over 65s.

Development of a person-centred dementia care approach

It used to be generally assumed within the realms of psychiatry that once people's dementia had progressed past a certain point they were beyond the reach of effective intervention by health professionals. As a result, the role of care providers was to offer shelter, warmth, nutrition and ensure that physical needs were met, in the belief that this was the most empathetic approach to care. However, as in all areas of nursing practice, there have been remarkable advances over the years in dementia care, both for the people living with dementia and their families, with a person-centred care approach now being widely used. The development of the person-centred care approach is widely attributed to Professor Thomas Kitwood, who was a psychologist in the late 1980s at the University of Bradford. He subsequently led the Bradford Dementia Group, which continues to be an institution of excellence with regard to dementia care.

Role of the district nurse

District mental health nurses working with older adults will often encounter people experiencing varying degrees of dementia in the community setting. The main role of the community nurse is to support the patient to try and help them remain as independent as possible and to promote their sense of wellbeing. To deliver person-centred dementia care effectively it is essential that the community nurse tries to perceive the world as the patient does. To achieve this it is necessary to form and maintain meaningful relationships both with the person and the person's family as they are a vital source of information on the patient's personal history, which is core to the delivery of a person-centred care approach. Formulating a personal history for the person experiencing dementia can be an extremely fulfilling experience as reminders of places, people and life events can bring joy to the person and their families (Figure 32.1).

Why is there a need for person-centred dementia care?

Although each individual's experience and journey of dementia is unique to them, Kitwood suggests that in order to maintain a sense of wellbeing, five main psychological needs must be met: comfort, attachment, inclusion, occupation and identity. It is recognised that most people are able to realise these needs independently much of the time and can compensate for any gaps, which allows an acceptable level of function. However, for patients experiencing dementia it becomes much more difficult to take the initiatives that would lead to their needs being met. The pattern of need will vary according to personality and life history and often the intensity of need is manifested as the person's dementia advances. This is one of the key reasons why a person-centred approach to care is needed. In this respect it is important to take account of a person's cultural background, as this could have a significant effect on what care is most appropriate and effective (Figure 32.2).

Supporting the person experiencing dementia and ensuring their sense of wellbeing is maintained is much more achievable in the person's own home, which is a familiar environment with familiar faces and routines. This support may become compromised when the person requires admission into a non-specialist care setting, including a general hospital.

Admission to the community and hospital sector

Because of the ageing population it is recognised that the incidence of dementia is rising. Subsequently, there is a higher instance of people experiencing dementia requiring care in the community, care home, hospice and hospital sectors, as physical compromise is highly associated with the ageing process.

A district nurse can play an important role here, including advocating for the person experiencing dementia and supporting the person and their families through the different care pathways, which may involve an admission to hospital or other settings. Acting as the person's advocate places the district nurse in a favourable position both to inform colleagues of the holistic needs of the person and offer advice and support accordingly (Table 32.1).

Evidence and research continue to recognise the need for an increased understanding of dementia care and this is supported by national and local stakeholders. Colleagues in non-specialist practice settings may experience a sense of failure and frustration when caring for this vulnerable client group, because of lack of specialist knowledge. This admission is a positive indicator for change. Increased knowledge and skills would improve staff competencies and promote confidence resulting in an improved patient experience and outcome.

33 Safeguarding

Helen Marshall, QN

Box 33.1   Key areas of district nurse assessment in the home environment.

Risk assessment	
Recognising signs of abuse	Carer assessment
Education of patient and family	Sharing knowledge

Box 33.3   The five principles of the Mental Capacity Act.

1 Every adult must be assumed to have capacity unless it is proven otherwise
2 All reasonable steps must be taken to assist the person to make a decision
3 Individuals have the right to make unwise decisions, even those others may consider eccentric
4 All actions on behalf of those who lack capacity must be in their 'best interests'
5 Any treatment should be done in the least restrictive manner of the person's basic rights and freedoms

Box 33.2   The six key principles of safeguarding.

Empowerment	• People should be supported to make their own decisions • If someone is unable to self-report abuse a district nurse should do this on their behalf
Prevention	• It is always better to be proactive than reactive where possible • The aim is too increase knowledge and education of both nurses and patients in order to recognise signs of abuse and respond as soon as possible
Proportionality	• A proportionate response to the risk presented must be taken • The higher the risk of harm and abuse, the higher the response rate needed
Protection	• An adult at risk may be unable to protect themselves against harm and abuse, and may be unable to report this • A district nurse should provide support and representation for those in greatest need through assessment and care planning
Partnership	• Working together for the good of the patient is always the gold standard for a district nurse • A safeguarding referral may involve a multi-agency response • Services have a statutory obligation to share information to share information and work together in order to protect adults at risk
Accountability	• A district nurse has a professional and statutory responsibility to be aware of safeguarding • A district nurse can demonstrate suitable accountability through robust documentation, which provides clear rationales for actions taken in order to keep both nurse and patient safe

Sources: Stuart Miles/Alamy Stock Photo, vepar5/123RF, pagadesign/Getty Images.

District Nursing at a Glance, First Edition. Edited by Matthew Bradby.
© 2022 John Wiley & Sons Ltd. Published 2022 by John Wiley & Sons Ltd.

Safeguarding is an integral component of every nurse's duty and should run through the core of district nursing practice in order reduce the risk of harm to people. Section 42 of the Care Act 2014 identifies that safeguarding duties apply when an adult has care and support needs and if, as a result of those needs, is unable to protect themselves from either the risk of, or experience of, abuse or neglect.

Adult safeguarding therefore means protecting an adult's right to live in safety, free from abuse and neglect. It is important that district nurses understand their role and responsibilities in relation to safeguarding and raise any concerns immediately. They should be able to identify who could be deemed an adult at risk, recognise potential abuse and be aware of procedures in place to report suspected abuse (Box 33.1).

Adult safeguarding is driven by six key principles, which the district nurse should be aware of and adhere to throughout their daily practice (Box 33.2). If a district nurse observes any abuse of a child during their care of an adult, they *must* report this to the local authority.

Types of abuse

Abuse can be categorised into types and these can occur in isolation, but often a person may experience more than one type. The types of abuse are physical, sexual, psychological, financial or material, discriminatory and organisational abuse, domestic abuse, modern slavery, neglect and acts of omission and self-neglect. Abuse may be a one-off event, or it can happen multiple times, affecting one or more people. A perpetrator may be a stranger, yet predominantly the perpetrator will be known to the individual and can be in a position of power and trust. It is important that district nurses are aware of what abuse can look like in order to identify and escalate in a timely manner.

Assessment

A thorough holistic assessment can aid practitioners to recognise and reduce the risk of abuse. However, district nurses should appreciate that people can lead complex lives, and being safe is only one of the things they want for themselves. Therefore, it should be established through a holistic assessment what 'being safe' means to them, and how this is best achieved. It is also important to take account of cultural differences, to treat these sensitively and if necessary take further advice. A district nurse should undertake risk assessments to ensure any risk identified is acted upon and minimised. A multidisciplinary meeting may also be considered when planning care. Safeguarding should be person-centred.

Making a referral

In order to achieve the best outcomes for patients, professionals must work together and create strong multi-agency partnerships. A district nurse may work with people from the health sector, local authority, police and many others. It is recommended that you thoroughly familiarise yourself with your organisation's policies and procedures that apply.

The local authority has the statutory responsibility to make enquiries or cause others to do so if it believes an adult is at risk of, or experiencing, abuse. If, as a district nurse, you suspect abuse or abuse has been disclosed to you, it is important not to ignore it. A referral is made by contacting the local authority where the incident happened and advising them exactly why you are concerned. It is vital to document your actions in order to demonstrate you have acted professionally and accountably. Findings from previous case reviews have shown that if people act upon their concerns sooner, serious harm may be prevented.

Carers and safeguarding

Being a carer can be an extremely rewarding role, yet at times it is noted to be stressful, and physically and mentally demanding. A district nurse should incorporate carers in their assessment of a patient, to indicate whether further support is required and to address the risk of carer breakdown. A carer may intentionally or unintentionally harm the adult they are caring for. Harm may be caused due to stress, carer breakdown, a lack of knowledge and training, or the escalating complexity and demands of the person they are caring for. The needs of an adult at risk should be addressed separately from the person alleged to be causing the harm, as both parties can be considered vulnerable.

The Mental Capacity Act 2005

The Mental Capacity Act (MCA) 2005 is statutory guidance in England and Wales, designed to protect and empower people to support them when making decisions if they have a diagnosed impairment of the mind or brain. In certain situations, the MCA enables practitioners such as a district nurse to make health-related decisions on a person's behalf if an assessment concludes they lack the mental capacity to make a decision themselves. This practice is called 'acting in best interests'. District nurses must follow and adhere to the five governing principles of the MCA (Box 33.3). It is important to note that mental capacity is always presumed unless a documented assessment demonstrates otherwise.

Section 44 of the MCA facilitates a criminal prosecution of those found guilty of ill treatment and wilful neglect of a person who lacks mental capacity.

Safeguarding is everyone's duty, and it should run through the core of every district nurse's practice in order to protect adults at risk.

34 Supporting carers

Julie Bliss, QN and Emma Lea, QN

Figure 34.1 Carers' Alert Thermometer (Edge Hill University). Source: Modified from Knighting, K., O'Brien, M.R., Roe, B. et al. (2015). Development of the carers' alert thermometer (CAT) to identify family carers struggling with caring for someone dying at home: a mixed method consensus study. *BMC Palliative Care* 14(1).

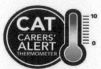

Carers' Alert Thermometer (CAT) V1.1

Edge Hill University

INSTRUCTIONS

Section 1 and 2 to be completed with the carer, ticking the risk level of any alerts to (a) the care being provided or (b) carers well-being;

L NO or LOW risk   **I** INTERMEDIATE risk   **H** HIGH risk

Section 3 circle the total number of **intermediate** (amber) and **high risk** (red) alerts on the thermometer;

Section 4 make a plan with the carer prioritising the top four alerts for action, and note the agreed appropriate action for the alerts identified;

Section 5 set a review date and person responsible for follow up. All questions to be revisited during a review to monitor for any change. It is recommended that monitoring and review dates be more frequent for carers with alerts which are considered 'HIGH' (red) or 'INTERMEDIATE' (amber).

Date CAT conducted:............................ **By (Staff name):**...**Tel:**.............................

SECTION 1: PLEASE COMPLETE THE DETAILS OF THE CARER & PERSON BEING CARED FOR

Carer's Name: .... *Relationship to cared for person:*..

Name of person caring for:.. *D.O.B.:*............................ *NHS No.:*....................

Address & Tel:..

GP of cared for person:..

Other key professional contact (if app):..

Carer address & Tel (if different):.. ....

SECTION 2: IDENTIFY & ASSESS THE NEEDS OF THE CARER

Discuss the following areas with the carer to identify any alerts requiring action. [x] = person being cared for e.g. husband or wife.

(A) CURRENT CARING SITUATION				**SECTION 3.** CIRCLE THE TOTAL NUMBER OF ALERTS ON THE THERMOMETER
Q1) Do you have any needs or concerns about caring for your [x]?	L	I	H	
Q2) Do you need any information about the condition your [x] has and how the care needed might change over time?	L	I	H	
Q3) Do you need any help to provide any of the physical or general daily care your [x] requires?	L	I	H	
Q4) Do you need any help to provide any emotional or spiritual care your [x] requires?	L	I	H	
Q5) Do you have a named person to call in an emergency or out-of-hours to discuss any concerns about your [x]?	L	I	H	
(B) CARER'S HEALTH AND WELL-BEING Q6) Do you feel involved in discussions and listened to by professionals about the care needed by [x]?	L	I	H	
Q7) Do you need any help or information about money or legal issues?	L	I	H	
Q8) Do you need a break from caring during the day or overnight?	L	I	H	
Q9) Do you need any help to balance your own needs with the demands of caring? *(e.g. attend own health appointments, social activities)*	L	I	H	
If appropriate include: Q10) Do you know your [x]'s wishes and preferences for EoL care? (If known, have they been written down and shared, e.g. advance care planning (ACP) doc?)	L	I	H	

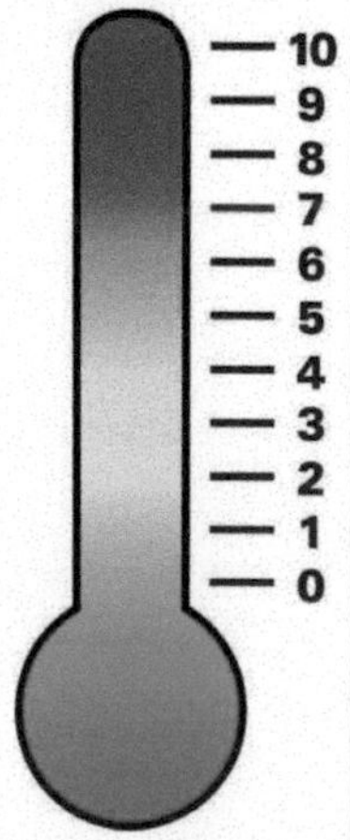

Thermometer scale: 10, 9, 8, 7, 6, 5, 4, 3, 2, 1, 0

Carers Alert Thermometer _ Version 1.1 **© Edge Hill University** Any correspondence to eprc@edgehill.ac.uk Further information is available at www.edgehill.ac.uk/carers

Figure 34.1 (Continued)

SUGGESTED NEXT STEPS Some general guidance is included below which can be amended by managers or senior clinicians of the service to help guide staff responses when conducting the CAT based on available local services and support.

Q1	If no needs raised with this opening question continue with the rest of the CAT.
Q2	Provide information to the carer if appropriate or refer to the appropriate professional.
Q3	Identify area of need, provide advice if appropriate. If needed, proceed to full assessment.
Q4	Discuss local & national sources of support for the carer & advise on routes of support for the patient e.g. GP
Q5	Identify if person cared for has a named professional for O-O-H contact. Advise on appropraite O-O-H support.
Q6	Discuss carer's concerns; if appropriate, liaise with appropriate health & social care professionals.
Q7	Provide information on local services e.g. local carer centre/ Citizen's Advice Bureau/Macmillan Cancer Support. If needed, proceed to full assessment.
Q8	Provide information about local respite care or sitting services. If needed, proceed to full assessment.
Q9	Provide information about local services and support e.g. carer centre. If needed, proceed to full assessment.
Q10	If appropriate, ask if they would like information on Advance Care Planning. If needed, proceed to full assessment.

SECTION 4: PLAN. Use this table to briefly note the details of each priority alert, any actions taken, and any next steps which have been agreed with the carer

Brief summary of needs identified by alerts (If there are several needs, ask the carer to "identify which one thing would help you most at this time?")	Any immediate action taken e.g. information clarified, verbal or written information given, referred to see other health care professional	Any next steps required? e.g. Referral to other services, speak to Team Leader/Manager for advice on next steps	Who is responsible for the next step or follow up?

SECTION 5: Date of next review:........................ with..

If possible, please give an indication of the GSF indicator stage of the person being cared for by circling the most appropriate stage:

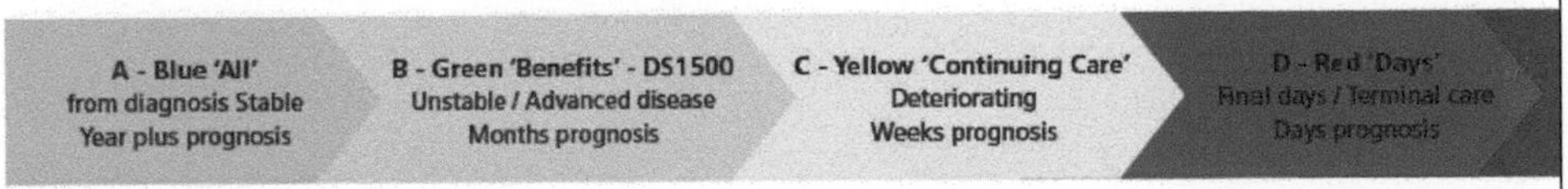

A - Blue 'All' from diagnosis Stable Year plus prognosis | B - Green 'Benefits' - DS1500 Unstable / Advanced disease Months prognosis | C - Yellow 'Continuing Care' Deteriorating Weeks prognosis | D - Red 'Days' Final days / Terminal care Days prognosis

Figure 34.2 Carers' Alert Thermometer – Guidance for Staff. Source: Based on Knighting, K., O'Brien, M.R., Roe, B. et al. (2015). Development of the carers' alert thermometer (CAT) to identify family carers struggling with caring for someone dying at home: a mixed method consensus study. *BMC Palliative Care* 14(1).

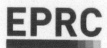 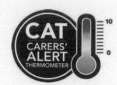 Edge Hill University

Carers Alert Thermometer - Guidance for staff

Thank you for your interest in using the CAT. Below are some short notes to guide your use of the CAT.

Eligibility Criteria

The CAT is designed to be used with:

➢ Unpaid carers who are supporting a patient at home during their expected last year of life; who are

➢ Adults aged 18+ years old.

Procedure

STEP 1: IDENTIFICATION

If you identify a carer who fulfils the eligibility criteria, introduce the idea of completing the CAT with them to identify any needs they may have in relation to their caring role and for their own well-being. If they wish to proceed, complete the CAT with them.

STEP 2 – COMPLETE THE CAT following the instructions on the front of the CAT.

Section 1 – complete the information section

Section 2 – Ask the questions, ticking the risk level of any alerts to **(a)** the care being provided or **(b)** carers well-being;

 NO or LOW risk   INTERMEDIATE risk   HIGH risk

Section 3 - circle the total number of **intermediate** (amber) and **high risk** (red) alerts on the thermometer;

Section 4 - make a plan with the carer, prioritising the top four alerts for action, and note the agreed appropriate action for the alerts identified;

Section 5 - set a review date and identify person responsible for follow up. All questions would be revisited during a review to monitor for any change. **It is recommended that monitoring and review dates are more frequent for carers with alerts which are considered 'INTERMEDIATE'** (amber) **or 'HIGH'** (red).

STEP 3 – IMMEDIATE ACTION

If any of the alerts can be supported immediately, such as provision of information or signposting to sources of support, these should be completed. All other alerts should be included in the action plan indicating the appropriate action and review date.

INFORMATION SOURCES

The provision of written information with sources of support for carers was highly valued by carers during the pilot of the CAT and is encouraged where possible. Local resources and information about local carer centres can be used where available. A directory of support available for carers, containing information for each region in the North West of England and national organisations, has been produced by Merseyside and Cheshire Cancer Network which can be accessed here http://www.mccn.nhs.uk/index.php/patients_cancer_help_and_support

CAT Research Team Contact Details

● If you would like more information about the study or have any questions or comments about completing the CAT please contact the team at eprc@edgehill.ac.uk or 01695 650941.

● There is also information available on the project website at www.edgehill.ac.uk/carers

● Please note this is for guidance about using the CAT, not advice on the next appropriate action in response to alerts.

District nurses must ensure that they identify individuals who are providing unpaid care and supporting individuals to stay at home. In order to support carers it is important to work in partnership with them, as well as with the patient and health and social care providers to meet the ongoing needs of both patient and carer.

The Carers Act 2014 strengthens the rights of carers and for the first time includes the right of carers to receive services. In addition the Children and Families Act 2014 sets out new duties, including the assessment of parent carers of children under 18 and young carers (Carers UK, 2014a).

The needs of carers

The Carers Trust has made a number of recommendations with regards to supporting carers that could be facilitated by the nurse directly or by referral on to the appropriate service. These include the following recommendations:

- Physical and mental health:
  - Physical healthcare check once per year by GP
  - All carers screened for depression once per year by GP
  - Effective methods for promoting wellbeing
- Training for carers:
  - Moving and handling
  - Managing challenging behaviour
- Planning for the future
  - Emergency care schemes can remove a great deal of worry for carers
- Recognition by health and social care professionals
  - Breaks for carers
  - Financial support.

With regard to financial support it is important that carers have information about what is available. In addition to carer's allowance, services and support accessed through personal budgets can be used to improve the carer–service user relationship. Although personal budgets have much to offer carers and the cared for person, local authority processes and paperwork can cause additional stress for carers (Larkin, 2015). The nurse and other members of the integrated team can assist by supporting the carers and cared for person in setting up a personal care package, utilising all skills within the team.

Partnership working

Partnership working with carers should recognise the caring context and carers' expertise to reduce the amount of conflicting information that carers receive, thereby reducing potential confusion and consequent frustration carers may experience (McPherson et al., 2014). An exploration of carers' experience of working with health and social care staff identified several important issues that the nurse needs to acknowledge in partnership working, including the following:

- Quality of care for the recipient: 'real' caring was important
- Knowledge exchange: carer perspectives must be valued
- One size does not fit all: the service needs to be flexible.

Assessment of carer needs

An understanding of the needs and challenges facing carers is helpful; however, it is important that the uniqueness of each carer and their circumstance is considered. One tool that can facilitate the assessment of individual carer need is the Carers' Alert Thermometer, which has been developed for use with adult carers who are supporting a person at home during end-of-life care (Knighting et al., 2015). The tool was developed by carers and professionals across health and social care settings and supports identification of needs in the present and future (Figures 34.1 and 34.2).

The National Institute for Health and Care Excellence (NICE) screening questions for depression provide a mechanism to identify carers who may be depressed. If the carer responds 'yes' to either of the following questions, further assessment should be undertaken using the Patient Health Questionnaire (PHQ-9)(http://patient.info/doctor/patient-health-questionnaire-phq-9).

- During the last month, have you often been bothered by feeling done, depressed or hopeless?
- During the last month, have you been often bothered by having little interest or pleasure in doing things?

Carers can also be encouraged to undertake self-assessment of their wellbeing using the NHS Choices website.

Summary

The document 'Supporting the health and wellbeing of adult carers' (Department of Health, 2014) identified a number of key actions that can also be applied to working with young carers. These actions provide a helpful *aide-memoire* when working in partnership with carers:

- Empower carers:
  - Ensure support systems help carers to live their own lives
  - Recognise each carer as the expert in providing care and support for another person
- Family-centred approaches to care:
  - Support and provide decision-making processes that focus on the health and wellbeing needs of the carer
- Partnership working within the changing health and social care agenda:
  - Recognise the core values of supporting carers
- Collaborative-working
  - Empower and optimise the health and wellbeing of carers
- Use informal support networks for carers, e.g. befriending, peer support and carers' organisations.

35 Supporting young carers and older carers

Julie Bliss, QN and Emma Lea, QN

Figure 35.1 Triangle of care. Source: Modified from Hannan R, Thompson R, Worthington A & Rooney P (2013). *The Triangle of Care Carers Included: A Guide to Best Practice for Dementia Care.* London: Carers Trust.

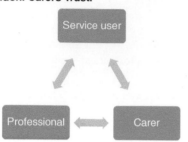

Figure 35.2 Carers UK.

Figure 35.3 Carers Trust.

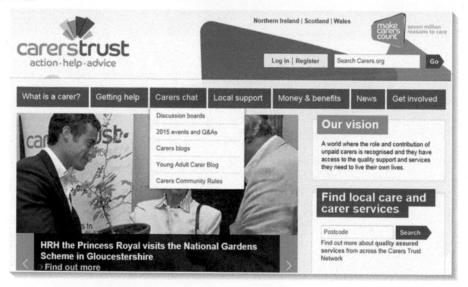

Figure 35.4 The Queen's Nursing Institute learning resource.

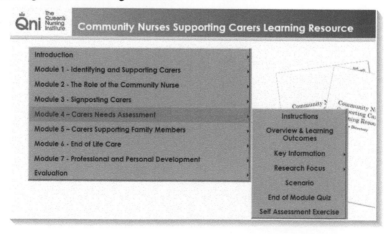

District Nursing at a Glance, First Edition. Edited by Matthew Bradby.
© 2022 John Wiley & Sons Ltd. Published 2022 by John Wiley & Sons Ltd.

Caring through the life course

It is estimated that around 10% of the UK population are carers. The number of people providing unpaid care has grown faster than the overall increase in the population and this trend is forecast to continue. Many people will find themselves new to a caring role at some point in their lives so it is important to ensure that people have the information and advice they need (Carers UK, 2014b).

For nurses, is important to help people to recognise that they are in a caring role, to help them access appropriate information and support. This is of particular importance for carers who are providing unpaid care for a close relative, as they may simply consider their role to be part of a family support network rather than that of unpaid carer. The role of carer is not restricted to adults but also includes young carers under the age of 18, many of whom are caring for a close relative who has a long-term condition, cancer, HIV, mental health condition or learning disability (McAndrew et al., 2012).

The impact on carers

Unpaid caring impacts upon the carer and the cared for person, potentially altering the dynamics of the relationship between the two. Over 7350 carers responded to the 2018 Carers UK Annual Survey, sharing their experiences and views of providing unpaid care (Carers UK, 2018). The survey identified that carers put their own health and wellbeing last, with 33% of respondents having been in a caring role for over 15 years. In addition, 37% reported that they were struggling to make ends meet, with 35% reporting that they had given up work to provide care. Approximately 72% of carers who responded to the survey had suffered mental ill health because of their caring role, with 61% reporting an impact on their physical health. Negative impacts on their health included:

- finding it difficult to get a good night's sleep;
- struggling to maintain a balanced diet;
- having experienced an injury or physical health deteriorated as a result of caring;
- feeling more stressed;
- feeling more anxious;
- suffering from depression as a result of their caring role.

Carers may not access financial support as a result of not having the right information. The reasons given by carers as to why they did not obtain financial support include:

- Not being given any advice regarding entitlement
- Not realising the financial support was available
- Thinking that they would not be entitled to financial support
- Being given the wrong advice
- Having problems applying for benefits (Carers UK, 2014).

As a result of this lack of understanding, over £1.1 billion of carers' allowance goes unclaimed every year, impacting upon quality of life for both carers and cared for people.

It is important to consider the experience of caring from the viewpoint of the carer. A study of informal carers' experiences of caring identified four themes with regards to caring for an older adult in the home (Rodger et al., 2015). Respondents emphasised the following:

- Your time is not your own
- Duty of care is very real
- Burden of caring can be considerable
- Support for informal carers, for example from family, friends and other organisations/individuals, is vital.

Young carers

In the same way as adult carers, young carers may experience a lack of leisure time; however, it is important to acknowledge that the individual experiences of young carers may be different. Young carers can experience isolation, stigma and bullying. Furthermore, there can be a lack of recognition of young carers' contribution to the family. Research exploring the experience of young carers identified several themes related to the caring role, including the following (McAndrew et al., 2012):

- Being excluded from decision-making
- Stuck in the here and now, ignoring the future: failure of others to understand the effect that caring has on young people's futures
- A hole in the net: lack of appropriate support for young carers
- Ensuring the 'hidden' is on the agenda: recognising who young carers are.

Health professionals should show young carers respect, not only as young people providing unpaid for care, but also as individuals within their own right. The carer, service user and professional should all be involved as equal partners in care delivery (Figure 35.1). Carers of all ages identify several key messages for healthcare professionals. These include the importance of considering the likelihood of partners undertaking reciprocal caring roles and the potential increasing frailty of older carers.

For young carers, it is important to support them if and when they transition to become adult carers (Department of Health, 2014). Resources available for unpaid carers and healthcare professionals include third-sector organisations such as Carers UK (www.carersuk.org) and the Carers Trust (www.carers.org). Both have websites which include helpful information and support (Figures 35.2 and 35.3).

Carers are a diverse group who should be considered as individuals with different strengths and needs, just as patients are treated as individuals. The Queen's Nursing Institute has bespoke learning materials for community nurses supporting carers on its website at https://www.qni.org.uk/nursing-in-the-community/supporting-carers/ (Figure 35.4). The resource includes a comprehensive resource directory with further links and information.

36 Palliative care

Vanessa Gibson, QN

Figure 36.1   A nurse and resident of a hospice.
Source: Courtesy of St Richard's Hospice.

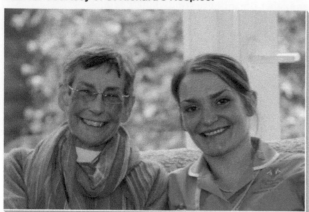

Figure 36.2   Therapy animals come in all shapes and sizes.

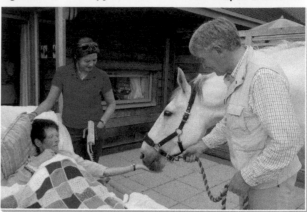

Figure 36.3   A nurse and a resident in a hospice setting.
Source: Courtesy of St Richard's Hospice.

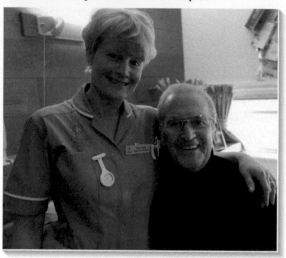

Figure 36.4   Palliative care in a a hospice setting.
Source: Courtesy of St Richard's Hospice.

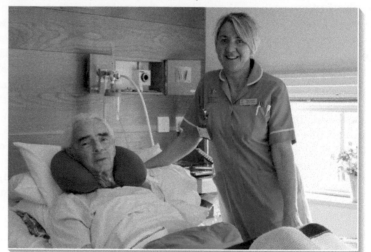

District Nursing at a Glance, First Edition. Edited by Matthew Bradby.
© 2022 John Wiley & Sons Ltd. Published 2022 by John Wiley & Sons Ltd.

By definition, palliative care is good nursing care. It is seeing beyond a diagnosis to see the whole person and what is important to them. The World Health Organization (2018) explains it as 'an approach that improves the quality of life of patients and their families facing the problem associated with life-threatening illness, through the prevention and relief of suffering by means of early identification and impeccable assessment and treatment of pain and other problems, physical, psychosocial and spiritual.'

Palliative care in practice – example

'Jan' has been diagnosed with advanced lung cancer. Minimal treatment is possible and none of the treatment offered will aim for cure; all is aimed at prolonging life and addressing her symptoms. But Jan is more than a woman with lung cancer. Jan is a mother, a sister and a daughter. She is a keen horsewoman and a self-employed landscape gardener. She has been working towards her retirement when she planned to hand over her business to her son and fulfil her own dreams of diving on the barrier reef in Australia. She is a spiritual person; although she does not practise a recognised religion she believes there is 'something more'. She is frightened and she is in pain.

Palliative care is recognising all that Jan is, seeing and responding to the whole person, controlling her pain, but also hearing her fears, regrets and concerns and helping her to find resolution where possible. It requires a careful use of team members to ensure Jan receives advice about benefits, and to ensure that her family and all people important to her are supported. The impact that the loss of her dreams, hobbies and future plans will have on Jan and her family must be recognised and helping Jan plan for the future and remain as well as possible, for as long as possible, is crucial to palliative care. This may sound overwhelming and, in truth, resolution is not always possible.

Central to palliative care is the notion of holistic care. As such, everyone involved in health and social care can provide palliative care. It is not simply the remit of hospices and specialist teams; palliative care is the foundation of all good care.

Any patient with a life-limiting diagnosis may require palliative care; they do not have to be at end of life or to have cancer. If we consider Jan again, she has just had her diagnosis and has treatment planned. She is not at end of life, but has multiple issues which need to be considered and, where possible, addressed. People with non-cancer diagnoses, for example kidney failure, heart failure or dementia, may well be in a similar position, in that cure is not possible and the diagnosed illness will have a significant impact on the patient's life.

Palliative care in district nursing

During palliative care, district nurses spend time with the patient, listening to their fears and concerns and agreeing a plan of action where possible (Figure 36.1). The plan of action will not be to achieve a cure. The plan of action will be to address key concerns that the patient and those important to them have. This may be something physical – for example, pain control. It could be social – for example, Jan may be too breathless to be able to get up and down her stairs at home. It may be much more psychological and spiritual – for example, Jan may be asking why she got cancer when she has lived a healthy and 'good' life. Finally, it may be very practical forward-planning – for example, thinking about where Jan would like to be cared for when she is approaching the end of life.

For some, a patient's plan of action may be very limited, and may be as simple as enabling a patient to see their pet again, giving them peace of mind that their pet is being well cared for (Figure 36.2). For others, it will be much more extensive.

Other palliative care services

Some peoples' palliative needs may be more complex. Pain may be difficult to control, or the level of psychological distress may be so high that additional specialist support is required. Specialist palliative services are available within hospital and community settings, and within specialist settings such as hospices. Staff working within specialist palliative care services will have normally undergone recognised specialist palliative care training. Specialist palliative care requires effective multidisciplinary working and coordination across a wide range of professions. This ensures that patients can achieve the best quality of life possible. Services work alongside the patient's own doctor and district nurse to enable the patient's symptoms to be controlled. This also allows support for the patient to be given with their chosen place of care; this could be their own home, nursing home, residential or care home, or for some patients mental health units, homeless hostels and prisons (Figures 36.3 and 36.4).

Although it is important to remember specialist teams exist, it is also important to remember that palliative care really is the remit of all staff involved within health and social care. The underlying principle is simply to see and work with the whole person, including those important to them.

Further information is available through the National Institute for Health and Care Excellence (www.nice.org.uk), the World Health Organization (www.who.int.en), Hospice UK (www.hospiceuk.org) and the National Council for Palliative Care (www.ncpc.org.uk).

Spirituality

Melanie Rogers, QN

Figure 37.1   Aspects of spirituality from the personal perspective. Source: Staffordshire University.

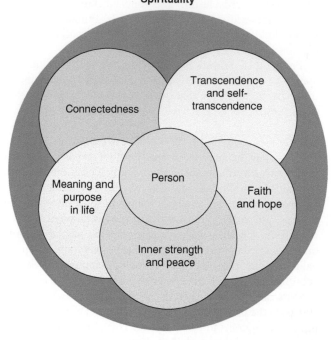

Spirituality

Connectedness

Transcendence and self-transcendence

Meaning and purpose in life

Person

Faith and hope

Inner strength and peace

Figure 37.2   Aspects of spirituality from a clinical perspective. Source: The Shrewsbury and Telford Hospital NHS Trust.

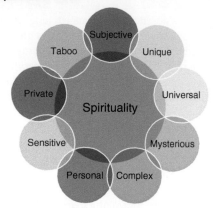

Subjective

Taboo

Unique

Private

Universal

Spirituality

Sensitive

Mysterious

Personal

Complex

Figure 37.3   A district nurse visiting a frail elderly person and family member.

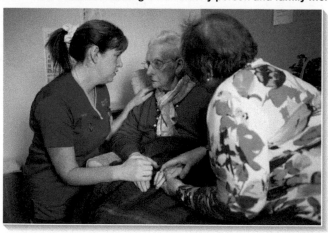

District Nursing at a Glance, First Edition. Edited by Matthew Bradby.

Spirituality is a fundamental part of holistic care that can easily be integrated into daily practice, yet it is often omitted due to confusion as to what it is and how to integrate it. Some people view spirituality as an emotive concept, some confuse spirituality and religion, and some adopt a wider perspective relating spirituality to concepts of hope, meaning and purpose in life. Others simply shy away from the subject as they are unsure what it actually means.

Spirituality is not the same as religion and is not necessarily wholly addressed if we have asked a patient about their religious beliefs. Spirituality is universal, individual and unique to each of us. For many people, spirituality may link to their relationships, connection with others, work, hobbies, nature, memory or faith. Supporting people in these areas is especially important when facing illness, mental health problems and crisis. Often when people become unwell and face personal trials the things that give hope, meaning and purpose are impacted significantly (Figure 37.1).

Holistic care in nursing must consider physical, social, economic, psychological and spiritual factors when assessing, planning and delivering care. Spirituality should be a way of practice, integrated through offering an open, caring and compassionate relationship to our patients. Many of us may not have seen this aspect of our care as 'spiritual', yet what we are doing in these interactions is showing that we value our patients, that we are listening to their concerns and that we want to support them to cope better with the issues they are facing (Figure 37.2).

Benefits of spirituality

Many studies have shown that addressing spirituality in nursing practice has the potential to improve patient outcomes, aid coping with illness and may reduce health costs by supporting patients with the underlying stress often prevalent in long-term conditions. As nurses striving to offer holistic care, we need to be aware that when patients are faced with illness, pain, vulnerability and distress they often look to spirituality. We are in the ideal place to listen to patients as they ask what can be deeply spiritual questions and invite us into their questioning. It is not uncommon for questions such as 'Why me?', 'What does this mean?', or 'How can I deal with this?' to be voiced. Being attentive to these questions can be openings to offer spiritual care and help patients to find some sense of hope, meaning and purpose during ill health. Simply being with a patient and listening attentively to these cues may be all that is needed.

If patients do not ask questions related to spirituality, it may be helpful to ask a few questions to open up the discussion. For example: 'How has this illness affected you/your relationships/ your activities/your work/your family?', 'Has your illness brought any special concerns with it?', 'Has it caused you to question things that you previously took for granted? What might help you to cope?' or 'What has being ill meant to you?'

In general, it is best to avoid questions beginning with 'why'. These are often perceived as critical or attributing blame. Other questions such as 'What is behind that?' can serve the same purpose in a less threatening way. These questions should lead to discussions about how the patient can be supported in addressing the needs identified, and these can then be included in the care plan (Figure 37.3).

Barriers to integrating spirituality into practice

A Royal College of Nursing study about spirituality found that one of the main barriers to integrating spirituality was confusion over what it really means. Other studies have found that nurses felt that it takes too much time, whilst others were concerned that the conversations may be too complex for them to manage. Seeing spirituality as a broad concept which links to hope, meaning and purpose should help nurses feel more comfortable about it. Equally, seeing it as the way we practice and not as an extra task helps to address the concerns about it taking too much time. Regarding complexity in conversations, nurses are in a prime position to build relationships with patients based on respect, and often develop a rapport where they can be honest and open in their interactions. Not having to have all the answers is something nurses are used to and, in reality, spirituality is not about having answers but just listening to patients as they share their concerns and questions.

Facilitators for integrating spirituality into practice

In order to feel comfortable with an individualised approach to spiritual care, cultural sensitivity and an ability to discern what is important to people is crucial. This is often different depending on a person's age, upbringing, values, culture and beliefs. Additionally, the person's hopes, expectations and ideas about meaning and purpose in life may differ to those of the nurse. It is important therefore that we be self-reflective, self-aware, and that we foster a non-judgemental attitude and be open with our patients. Listening has been shown to be a key feature of spiritual care; simply allowing a person to tell their own story and listening empathetically may give them an opportunity to discuss what illness means for them and to understand how it may be disrupting their sense of purpose in life.

38 Bereavement

Julia Fairhall, QN

Figure 38.1 Taking time to discuss a person's health and care is a key part of the District Nursing role. Courtesy of Matthew Peasey.

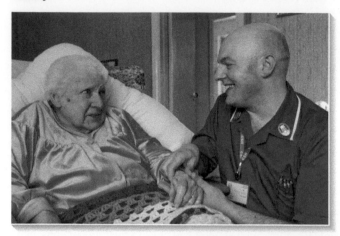

Figure 38.2 The Kübler-Ross grief cycle.

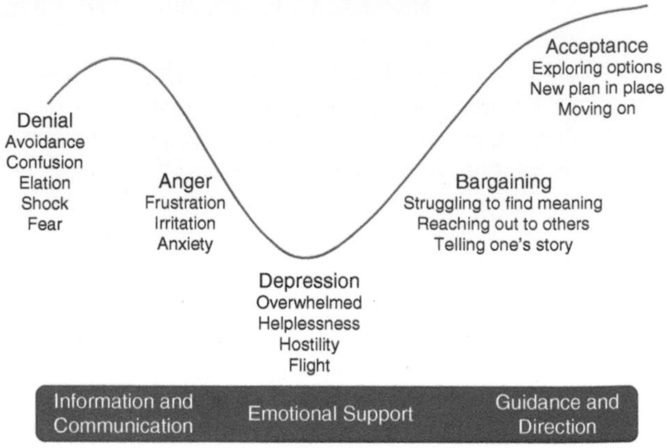

Denial
Avoidance
Confusion
Elation
Shock
Fear
Anger
Frustration
Irritation
Anxiety
Depression
Overwhelmed
Helplessness
Hostility
Flight
Bargaining
Struggling to find meaning
Reaching out to others
Telling one's story
Acceptance
Exploring options
New plan in place
Moving on
Information and Communication
Emotional Support
Guidance and Direction

Figure 38.3 Good communication is essential to building relationships in the home environment.

District Nursing at a Glance, First Edition. Edited by Matthew Bradby.

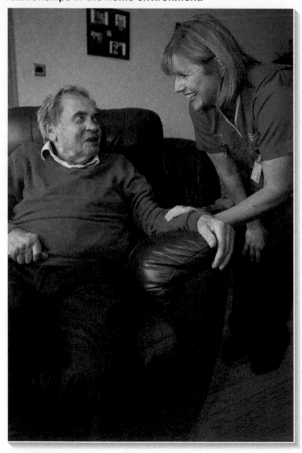

Death is a natural part of our life cycle, but dealing with death and the loss of a loved one can be a very distressing experience. End-of-life and bereavement care provided by district nurses often remains engraved on the memories of bereaved relatives. The relationship between the district nurse, the patient and their families is paramount in providing high-quality end-of-life care. End-of-life care includes bereavement care and district nurses have a fundamental role in supporting families with their bereavement.

Family bereavement

For families, bereavement is an extremely difficult time; many will have supported their loved ones to remain at home with regular visits from district nursing team members. During illness, they have had to cope with their loved one's physical, emotional, social and spiritual needs becoming more complex, and often will have had to coordinate care delivery by visiting professionals (Figure 38.1). Relatives will have been part of difficult conversations and experienced an intense emotional journey, often forgoing their own personal needs, with the support they require being unrecognised. For some families, as well as coping with the loss of a loved one, they may also have to deal with loss of the caring role that had become a way of life. For some, there will be experiences of relief, but also a sense of guilt for experiencing that emotion, and feelings of exhaustion and loneliness.

Role of the district nurse in bereavement care

The role of the district nurse involves holistic assessment of both the patient and those most important to the patient to develop a unique individualised care package. This involves collaborating with multidisciplinary teams and health professionals, and liaising and sourcing relevant care and support. It encompasses patients' physical, social, psychosocial, emotional, cultural and religious needs.

It is imperative during the assessment process that the district nurse enquires about specific cultures and customs of caring for the dying and bereavement practices that pertain to an individual's and family's cultural beliefs. Beliefs, rituals and traditions specific to a person's culture can provide familiarity and assurance during a time that is often difficult and confusing. These customs are fundamental information for the district nurse, as they can also provide directions that assist with structure at the time surrounding death.

The district nurse's communication and assessment skills are also crucial in supporting families through bereavement. When death is anticipated, helping those closest to the patient with open, transparent communication can assist with the grieving process.

Listening is a key skill. With proficient training, district nurses are skilled practitioners who are able to decipher the grieving process and recognise that grief is not a neat process. Part of the district nurse's role is to acknowledge the normality of the stages of grief and recognise, as unique individuals, people will move in and out of stages within their own journey pace. The Kübler-Ross model identifies the five stages of grieving, and can be applied to any situation (Figure 38.2).

The model discusses the first stage as denial, a disbelief of the event, then anger by what has happened. People describe resenting the relative they have lost for leaving them. Thirdly bargaining, feelings of helplessness and vulnerability are often seen as a need to regain control. Depression is the next stage and finally acceptance of the situation. However, individuals will not follow this model perfectly and can bounce between stages, sometimes becoming trapped within one phase. District nurses need the ability to recognise 'what grief looks like' and to acknowledge when families demonstrate emotions and behaviours that require signposting to more specialist services.

There are no time limits and no set patterns of behaviours or emotions. It is widely recognised that the district nurse's compassion and sensitivity throughout the end-of-life care journey can impact positively on the grieving process to enable individuals, with time, not to forget their loved ones but to manage their daily lives. If the patient and relatives have a poor experience of care and support, it can have lasting negative impact on their grieving and coping mechanisms. Getting the care right is fundamental.

Most district nursing services will provide at least one bereavement visit to the family following the funeral. This visit is a time to assess and reflect with the family on how they are managing. It also gives families the opportunity to discuss the care, the journey and emotions they are experiencing. It allows the district nurse to reinforce the positivity and care the family gave to the patient (Figure 38.3). To support families at this stage, it is important that the district nurse builds a trusting relationship with family members. The family will not always remember the individual nurse or the words that are shared but will always remember how the nurse made them feel.

Bereavement help for district nurses

The death of patients does have a bearing on district nurses and can impact on the individual, their working environment and even influence their home lives. Employing organisations support staff with clinical supervision on a regular basis. Educational opportunities exist to develop a sound knowledge of the theory of grief and its processes; advanced communication skills are key to developing coping strategies and resilience. District nurses also create informal support networks to assist their colleagues in dealing with bereavement.

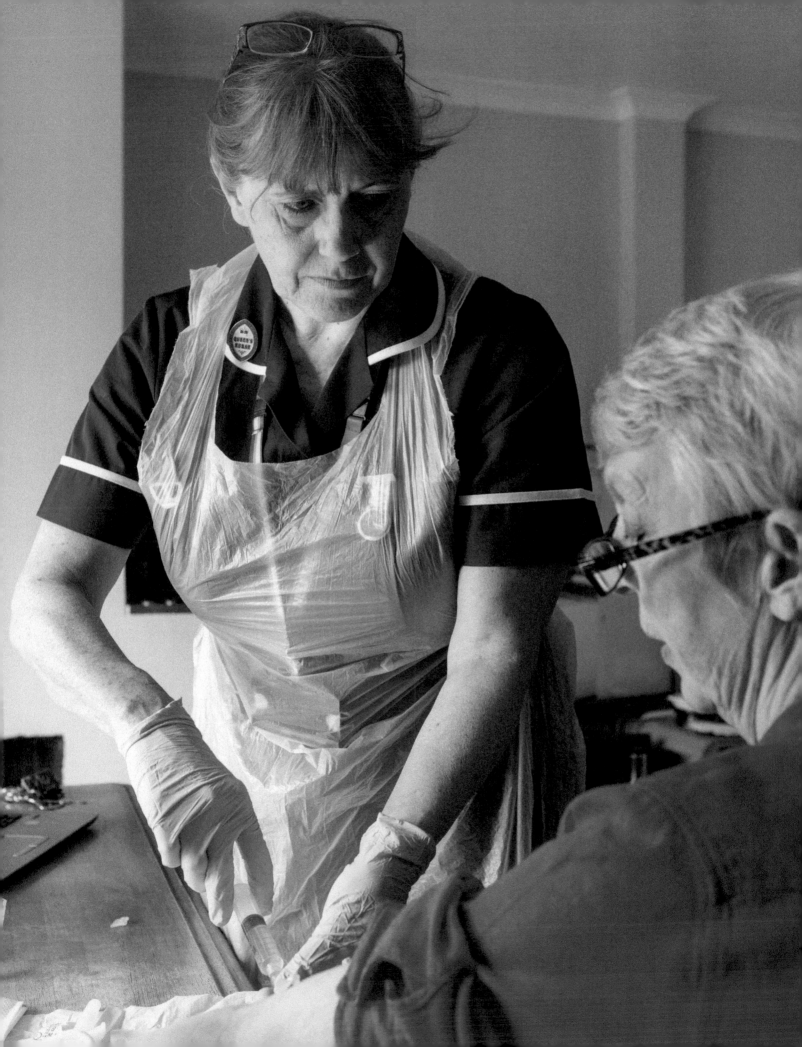

Physical and mental health in the community

Part 5

Chapters

39 Holistic nursing assessment in the community

Emma Brodie, QN

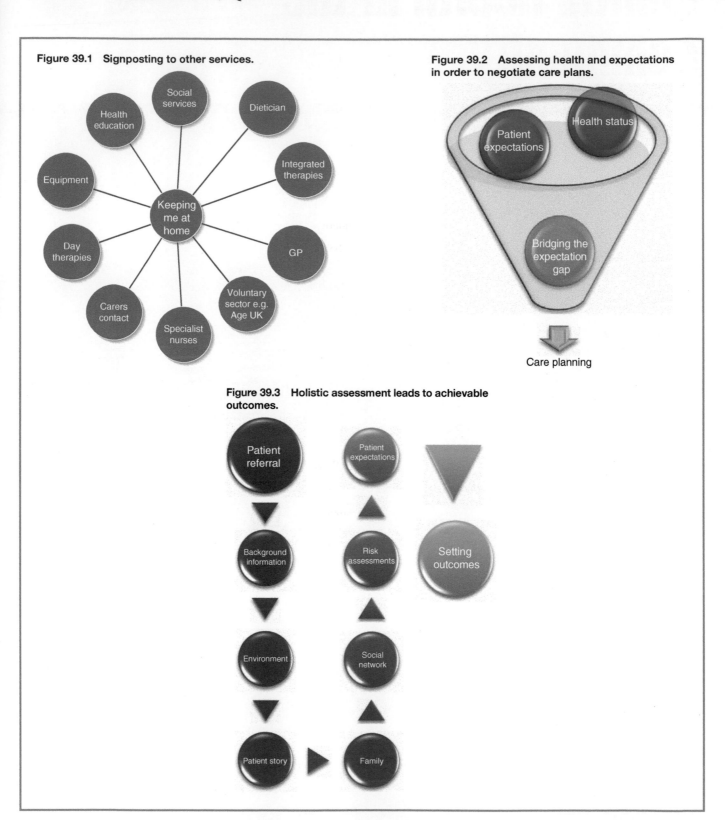

Figure 39.1 Signposting to other services.

- Social services
- Health education
- Dietician
- Equipment
- Integrated therapies
- Keeping me at home
- Day therapies
- GP
- Carers contact
- Voluntary sector e.g. Age UK
- Specialist nurses

Figure 39.2 Assessing health and expectations in order to negotiate care plans.

- Patient expectations
- Health status
- Bridging the expectation gap

Care planning

Figure 39.3 Holistic assessment leads to achievable outcomes.

- Patient referral
- Patient expectations
- Background information
- Risk assessments
- Setting outcomes
- Environment
- Social network
- Patient story
- Family

District Nursing at a Glance, First Edition. Edited by Matthew Bradby.
© 2022 John Wiley & Sons Ltd. Published 2022 by John Wiley & Sons Ltd.

The physical effects of chronic and acute periods of ill health can have significant implications for a person's quality of life. The provision of a holistic and flexible health needs assessment is therefore a vital role in district nursing. The assessment process allows the patient to have protected one-to-one time with the nurse, to discuss the impact of illness on their lifestyle, wellbeing and future plans.

Establishing the individual's abilities, both pre-illness and currently, is an important aspect of the assessment and allows for identification of present and future risks, such as the potential for pressure ulcer development, malnutrition or falls. The process provides a platform for health education, multidisciplinary support and preventative care planning and has the potential to reduce future hospital admissions. It is for this reason that assessment is both complex, dynamic and extremely important.

Environment

The home environment is very different to the largely controlled and clinical environment of a hospital ward. Most district nurses are habituated to chaotic or cluttered homes, poorly controlled pets, loud televisions and couples arguing during their visit. It must be remembered that the community nurse is a guest in the home and can request, but not dictate, as to the environment provided. Although an untidy house may indicate that someone is struggling to cope, for others it may just be the norm. The ability to observe, listen and question in a sensitive, non-judgemental and open manner is fundamental.

The majority of people live in homes that are not designed to meet the needs of those with altered or ill health. Simple tasks that are usually taken for granted, for example going up stairs to the toilet or to bed, may prove impossible or place someone at risk of falls and injury. Similarly, sleeping downstairs in a chair could result in sustaining pressure damage. Through assessing both the environment and how the person is coping, the nurse is ideally placed to provide suggestions or equipment and to signpost to other members of the multidisciplinary team, such as physiotherapy and occupational therapy (Figure 39.1).

Family and culture

In an increasingly diverse population, nurses need to have an underlying knowledge of the communities in which they work. Cultural, economic and social diversity all impact on day-to-day living and the health choices made by individuals. The assessment process must, therefore, revolve around establishing the beliefs, practices and expectations held by patients and their families. As the term 'community' indicates, people do not live in isolation and it is good practice to establish, within the assessment, who and what are most important to the patient. If you are recommending total bed rest to someone who has tickets to an event they have been looking forward to for months, they are unlikely to comply with the plan. It would be better to discover this at the time of your assessment, so that an alternative treatment pathway may be suggested.

This is particularly relevant where other people live within the property, because care plans may affect them too. If, for example, there is a need for a pressure relief mattress and it is a double bed, will the patient's partner be willing to sleep on it? Consideration should also be given to whether the patient is a carer themselves, and whether additional support may be needed during the period of ill health. This may be relevant if there are young children or an elderly dependent living in the property. Once identified, the nurse can direct the family to appropriate services such as social workers, school nurses, and health visitors.

Communication

The gathering of information should not be an interrogation or tick box exercise; the questions asked must be relevant to that individual and where possible led by them. This is the essence of personalised care.

Once home from hospital, the implications of living with a long-term health impairment become reality. Nurses should not shy away from difficult conversations and, with good communication skills, it is possible to create an environment in which the person may feel confident to ask questions or express worries. One example would be the approach taken to altered body image, such as the formation of a colostomy, by asking, 'You have been through a big change; how is your family coping?' This indicates that the nurse is willing to have that discussion, but also allows the patient to give a generic answer if they do not wish to divulge personal information.

Future plans and expectations

A holistic assessment allows the nurse to ascertain the level of understanding that someone has about their condition and what support they may need to return to wellness, or to adjust to new circumstances. Once individual health outcomes have been identified, realistic care plans can be negotiated and implemented (Figure 39.2). The patient and nurse may only have face-to-face contact a couple of times a week and there is an increased chance of concordance if the individual's opinions have formed part of the decision-making process.

Because the district nurse is in the position of offering patients an assessment that encompasses all facets of living with illness (Figure 39.3), it is not unusual for the district nurse to become the key worker within the multidisciplinary team. If done well, it also provides a platform for care planning and support of the patient throughout their journey.

40 Baseline observations

Lucy Stewart, QN

Figure 40.1 Taking baseline observations in the home. Source: Lucy Stewart.

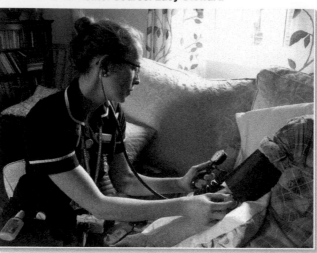

Figure 40.2 Heart rate (beats per minute).

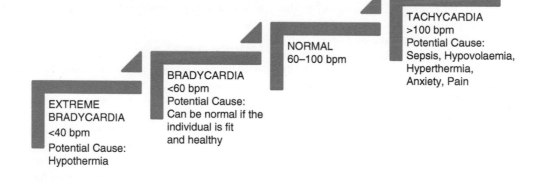

EXTREME BRADYCARDIA
<40 bpm
Potential Cause:
Hypothermia

BRADYCARDIA
<60 bpm
Potential Cause:
Can be normal if the individual is fit and healthy

NORMAL
60–100 bpm

TACHYCARDIA
>100 bpm
Potential Cause:
Sepsis, Hypovolaemia,
Hyperthermia,
Anxiety, Pain

Figure 40.3 The six R's.

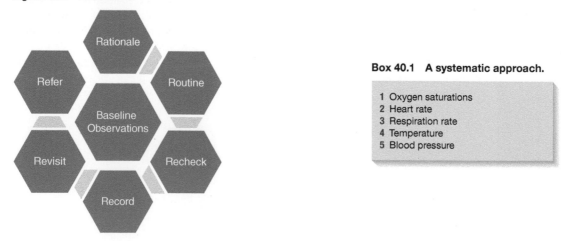

Rationale

Refer

Routine

Baseline Observations

Revisit

Recheck

Record

Box 40.1 A systematic approach.

1 Oxygen saturations
2 Heart rate
3 Respiration rate
4 Temperature
5 Blood pressure

District Nursing at a Glance, First Edition. Edited by Matthew Bradby.
© 2022 John Wiley & Sons Ltd. Published 2022 by John Wiley & Sons Ltd.

Vital signs or baseline observations are the least invasive way of checking a person's level of physical functioning. Normal observations change with age, weight, gender, exercise tolerance and physical condition. Heart rate (HR), respiration rate (RR), blood pressure (BP), temperature and oxygen saturation levels (SpO_2) are a vital source of information (Box 40.1). Used in combination, they can alert the nurse to a potential problem and steps can be taken to deal with this condition before it becomes worse or even life threatening. The challenge comes with making those observations standard and meaningful. One of the biggest challenges is that the home environment is far from clinical (Figure 40.1).

By using one's senses, an assessment can be made just by sight, smell, hearing, or by touching the patient. Elevated RR can be identified if the patient needs to sit forward in order to open their airways, if you can hear a chest wheeze or if the patient struggles to have a conversation. With pyrexia, the skin appearing flushed or feeling hot to the touch are indicative. For a low SpO2, discoloured peripheries such as lips or nose may be seen. In practice, it is often these symptoms that are noticed first, which then prompts the need to complete a full set of baseline observations.

Anyone who takes baseline observations should be aware of the normal physiological parameters. Establishing an oxygen saturation level is dependent on a person's peripheral circulation and is therefore susceptible to error. The pulse detection facility can be inaccurate due to movements such as shivering. Patients with a diagnosis of chronic respiratory disease generally function with a lower oxygen saturation level, often below 94% on room air. For those without this diagnosis a reading of 92–94% is a cause of concern and less than 92% could be serious.

It is not uncommon in the community – particularly among an ageing population – that an irregular heart rate is detected on palpation. Establishing if the rhythm is regular or irregular can be useful as an indication of electrical conduction problems in the heart, such as atrial fibrillation. Determining this irregularity can be difficult at first, but it is a skill that becomes easier with experience. If an irregularity is detected, it is important to ask the patient whether this is new or existing (Figure 40.2).

Not all patients presenting with respiratory symptoms have respiratory problems. Breathlessness can be a sign of cardiac difficulty too. RR is the most important and sensitive indicator that a person is developing a critical illness and a rise or fall in RR is the first physiological observation to change. A normal RR in an adult is 12–20 breaths per minute.

Blood pressure (BP) varies according to circumstances such as age, time of day, level of anxiety, physical activity, pain and disease processes (Medicines and Healthcare Regulatory Authority, 2013). These factors should be considered when interpreting recordings. A BP can be taken 30 minutes after food or exercise. If the BP needs to be repeated using the same arm, waiting 12 minutes will allow the circulation to return fully. When a patient reports fainting episodes, repeated falls or dizziness, a lying and standing BP is useful, as this could be postural hypotension. A person needs to stand for approximately one minute before a standing reading is taken. The Medicines and Healthcare Regulatory Authority provide a useful summary in the document 'Measuring blood pressure: top 10 tips' (MHRA, 2013).

Caution is advised in the use of automated devices when taking a BP, as the machine can fail to obtain a reading or give unreliable results in patients experiencing muscle tremors, weak pulse or low BP due to shock. Therefore, it is best practice to use a stethoscope and manual sphygmomanometer with the correct-sized cuff, with the patient's arm supported and their legs uncrossed to maintain accuracy. The equipment should ideally be at room temperature.

When making a holistic assessment, consideration should be given of a person's temperature. Wearing multiple layers of clothing, central heating and the time of year are all external factors that can influence a temperature reading and the reading may not necessarily reflect the body's core temperature.

Any deterioration due to infection can lead to the risk of suspected sepsis, where the body 'overacts' in its immune response and starts to inwardly damage its organs. Sepsis may just present as a person being very unwell or showing changes in their behaviour, rather than with a fever as you would expect. Early recognition is vital as this is life threatening but reversible if detected and treated early. Higher risk patients include the very young and old, those post-operative, immunosuppressed, or with indwelling catheters/lines, and those who inject drugs or sustain skin damage. The NICE guidelines on 'Sepsis: recognition, diagnosis and early management' (NICE, 2017) should be studied as there are risk-stratification tools which can help you to grade the severity of the patient in front of you, make sense of the baseline observations you have taken and decide on the urgent action required. Ultimately, if sepsis is suspected dial 999 without delay.

Safety netting

Some patients live with family members, but many live alone and a pendant alarm may be their only means of obtaining emergency assistance. The patient and any family members will need to be given verbal and written advice on 'what to do if …' whenever there are concerns with any clinical findings. This advice must always be documented in the patient's notes.

A district nurse is a gatherer of information and a GP will often require a series of observations, which is more useful in evaluating the person's condition than a single set of measures. After review, further investigations such as blood tests, ECG or X-rays may be required. Any element of risk should be assessed appropriately, documented and discussed with the GP/senior nurse (Figure 40.3).

Patients are often discharged from hospital to their own home very soon after surgery or other acute episodes to complete their recovery. The observations taken on the first contact may not necessarily be the person's own normal range, as they may still be unwell. Dependent on the clinical findings, a patient may need readmission, which is why it is so important to complete a routine set of baseline observations when first visiting.

41 Long-term conditions and co-morbidities

Lorraine Smith, QN

Figure 41.1 Examples of some common long-term conditions.

Hypertension Chronic Obstructive Pulmonary Disease
Chronic Heart Disease Heart Failure Cystic Fibrosis
Obesity Stroke End-of-Life
Dementia Asthma Depression

Figure 41.2 Disease pyramid.

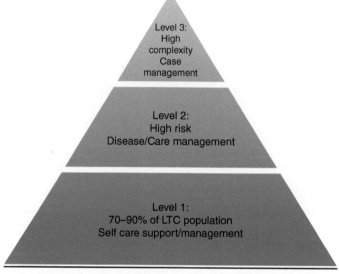

Level 3:
High complexity
Case management

Level 2:
High risk
Disease/Care management

Level 1:
70–90% of LTC population
Self care support/management

Figure 41.3 The NHS and Social Care Long Term Conditions model.

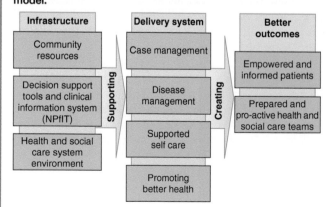

Figure 41.4 Self-management and self-care.

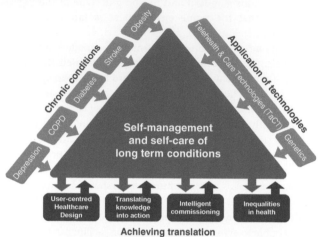

Figure 41.5 House of care.

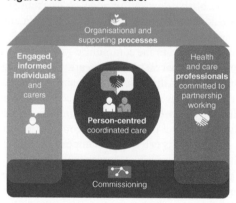

Figure 41.6 Long-term conditions and mental health.

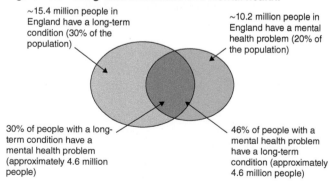

~15.4 million people in England have a long-term condition (30% of the population)

~10.2 million people in England have a mental health problem (20% of the population)

30% of people with a long-term condition have a mental health problem (approximately 4.6 million people)

46% of people with a mental health problem have a long-term condition (approximately 4.6 million people)

District Nursing at a Glance, First Edition. Edited by Matthew Bradby.
© 2022 John Wiley & Sons Ltd. Published 2022 by John Wiley & Sons Ltd.

The phrase 'long-term conditions' covers a range of diseases such as diabetes, chronic obstructive pulmonary disease (COPD), arthritis, hypertension, and dementia – diseases for which there is no cure. Co-morbidity is the presence of one or more diseases co-occurring with a primary disease or disorder. Co-morbidity can have an impact on increased hospital admissions and length of stay, and can have a major impact on health service resources (Figure 41.1).

There are currently estimated to be 15.4 million people in England with a long-term condition (LTC). This is predicted to rise to 18 million by 2025 because, due to an ageing population, there will be 42% more people in England aged 65 or over. The management of LTCs should be proactive, holistic, preventive and patient centred. Effective management, change of lifestyle, and rehabilitation can all improve a person's quality of life when living with an LTC.

Disease pyramid

The disease pyramid model acknowledges that people affected, or potentially affected, by LTCs have differing and complex needs (Figure 41.2). Level 1 refers to 70–80% of the population that self-manage their own condition, and may require advice on health promotion. Level 2 comprises those with a disease-specific unstable LTC. This is the level at which community nurses are mostly likely to be involved. Level 3 patients are those with highly complex multiple conditions that require intensive case management.

Self-management

There is good evidence that providing effective management for people with LTCs can improve their quality of life. Person-centred services for people with LTCs should be coordinated, support self-management, engage people in decisions, provide effective prevention and early diagnosis in conjunction with emotional, psychological, and practical support to provide the best outcomes. As a district nurse your role will concern health education and promotion. You will be involved in signposting patients to the most appropriate source of information and assisting them in making the right choices (Figures 41.3 and 41.4).

Integrated health and social care planning

The importance of LTC management is to provide the holistic assessment which identifies and addresses health and social care needs. It is important to ensure that a community-based multidisciplinary support mechanism is in place to address those needs, recognising the progressive nature of LTCs. This allows a seamless approach between professionals to include appropriate sharing of information. Building relationships with the hospital sector during an admission or hospital appointments helps to provide consistency of care between hospital and primary care, to allow a smooth transition and effective ongoing management.

House of care

Personalised care planning is at the centre of the house (Figure 41.5). This is a collaborative process designed to bring together the perspectives and expertise of both the individual and the professional(s) involved in providing care. It allows for tailored personal support to develop the confidence and competence needed for effective self-management. The two side walls of the house – engaged, informed patients and healthcare professionals – are equally important. Patients may need extra encouragement to participate in a more active way than they are used to, so consideration needs to be given to preparing them for self-management. District nurses need to understand this new way of working, valuing the contribution that each person can bring to their care and developing the skills to support self-management. Partnership working also extends to colleagues, as care for people with LTCs will increasingly be provided by multidisciplinary teams, both within general practice but also linking with wider community, social care and specialist staff. The roof of the house represents the robust organisational systems that are essential to ensure reliable systems for identifying and contacting patients with LTCs, flexible appointment systems that support linked contacts and allow for longer consultations when necessary, and record systems to document and share care plans and for monitoring outcomes. All this requires the firm foundation of a responsive local commissioning system. Care planning itself – and the systems and training needed to support it – must be explicitly commissioned: the relationship with community groups and services must be developed and a robust measurement system must be put in place.

Mental health

More than 4 million people in the UK have an LTC and mental health issues (Figure 41.6). Evidence demonstrates that those with LTCs are two or three times more likely to develop mental ill health. People with two or more LTCs are seven times more likely to experience depression than those without an LTC.

Providing high-quality care for all patients means that we must close the health gap between people with mental health problems and the population as a whole. Addressing mental health and psychological needs will improve the quality of life for the individual, and may reduce the impact and costs related to physical LTCs (e.g. from chest pain, chronic obstructive pulmonary disease and diabetes). The cost of managing a patient with diabetes and co-morbid depression is 4.5 times higher than the cost of managing a patient with diabetes alone. Therefore, people must be assessed and treated holistically for their health problems, rather than providing separate services for physical and mental disorders. Psychological therapies are crucial to this to provide the best outcomes for the patient.

42 Hydration

Alice Chingwaru, QN

Figure 42.1   Proper hydration is vital to physical and mental health.

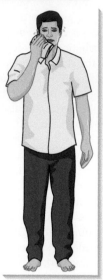

Figure 42.2   Ensure water is always available.

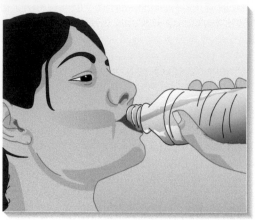

Figure 42.3   A poster illustrating a QNI-funded project, 'Water for Wellbeing', led by Carolyn Lindsay.

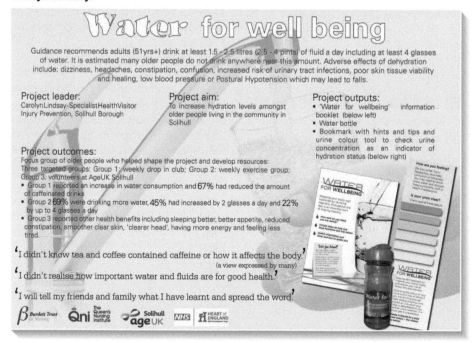

Water is crucial to all life and is the most abundant inorganic compound found in living material. This chapter will discuss the importance of water in health, homeostatic imbalances and nursing considerations for people presenting with dehydration (where the body loses more fluid than is taken in). Between 1 and 2 litres of fluid are lost in the form of urine from the kidneys each day and it is advised to drink six to eight glasses of fluid a day to replace the lost volume. The amount will vary according to individual characteristics and environmental factors (Figure 42.1).

The uses of water in the body

Water performs various functions in the body:

- *Shock absorber*: Water serves to form a resilient cushion around joints and certain body organs, helping to protect them from physical trauma. The cerebrospinal fluid surrounding the brain exemplifies water's cushioning role.
- *Thermo-regulator*: Water has a high heat capacity, absorbing relatively large amounts of energy before changing temperature itself. This helps the body to maintain a core temperature of between 36 and 37.5 degrees Celsius, regardless of sudden changes in temperature caused by external conditions. When a person is hot, water evaporates from the skin through perspiration, removing large amounts of heat from the body by an efficient cooling system of vaporisation. Efficient thermoregulation requires that a person is well hydrated.
- *Reactant*: In many chemical and metabolic processes, such as in digestion, foods are broken down to their building blocks by adding a water molecule to each chemical bond to be broken. It is therefore advocated that people drink water before meals to facilitate good digestion.
- *Transport medium*: Water is a component flowing in the circulatory, lymphatic and cerebral spinal systems. As a solvent, it is the essential medium to transport nutrients and oxygen into the cells whilst removing toxins and waste products for elimination through the kidneys, lungs, skin and gastrointestinal tract. Smoking, eating salty, fatty foods or foods high in cholesterol affect the transportation and diffusion of chemicals in and out of cells, as well as the ability to eliminate toxins.

Fluid and electrolyte balance

The body contains a variety of ions, or electrolytes, which perform a variety of functions. All of the ions contribute to the osmotic balance that controls the movement of water between cells and their environment. In terms of body functioning, six electrolytes are most important: sodium, potassium, chloride, bicarbonate, calcium and phosphate. They aid in nerve excitability, endocrine secretion and membrane permeability, and control the movement of fluids and body hydration levels. These ions enter the body via food and fluids through the digestive tract; excretion occurs mainly through the kidneys, with lesser amounts lost in sweat and in faeces.

The principal abnormalities of water balance in the body are dehydration, hypotonic dehydration and oedema. This chapter will concentrate on dehydration, defined as a loss of more than 3% of body weight associated with water, and electrolyte disturbance from water or sodium imbalance. People eating a typical Western diet, which is very high in table salt (sodium chloride, NaCl), routinely take in 130–160 mmol/day of sodium; however, humans require only 1–2 mmol/day. Elevated sodium levels in the body rapidly result in thirst, and indicate that additional water intake is needed (Figure 42.2).

Mild to moderate dehydration can exacerbate numerous health conditions and cause symptoms including light-headedness, dizziness, dry mouth, headaches, fatigue, asthma and allergies, skin disorders, joint pain, constipation, hypertension, digestive disorders, urinary tract infections and weight gain. Dehydration is a frequent cause of hospitalisation for infants, children and elderly adults as they are at increased risk of becoming dehydrated (Figure 42.3).

Severe dehydration can result from trauma, haemorrhage, severe burns, prolonged diarrhoea and vomiting, profuse sweating, fever, water deprivation, high alcohol intake and diuretic misuse. Endocrine disorders such as diabetes mellitus and diabetes insipidus can also cause dehydration. Prolonged dehydration leads to weight loss, fever and mental confusion. If unresolved, severe electrolyte dilution can lead to severe metabolic disturbance, nausea, vomiting, cramping of muscles and cerebral oedema. Uncorrected cerebral oedema leads to disorientation, convulsions, coma and death.

Nursing considerations for the client presenting with dehydration

Treatment options depend on the severity of dehydration. The district nurse may be ask to conduct a holistic assessment of the client including:

- Taking baseline vital signs, such as blood pressure, pulse, temperature, noting peripheral pulses, weight and urinalysis
- Monitoring blood pressure and invasive haemodynamic parameters
- Strictly monitoring fluid input and output observing physical properties of the urine
- Assessing skin turgor, mucous membranes and complaints of thirst
- Assessing neurological status
- Offering oral hydration therapy
- Administering intravenous fluids if indicated and monitoring effects
- Reviewing patient's medication, especially drugs with high sodium content
- Weighing the client daily
- Listening to the client to find out how they are feeling
- Providing health promotion messages on drinking enough water, low sodium nutritional intake and advocating lifestyle changes.

Daily evaluation is necessary, comparing client's minimum fluid requirements against recorded output. True nursing care that makes a difference is about reading and interpreting symptoms to help people recover quickly from their illness. Understanding water and its many uses is essential to nursing a person with dehydration back to health, regardless of their age.

43 Nutrition in the community setting including enteral feeding

Alison Burton Shepherd, QN and Susan Dunajewski, QN

Figure 43.1 The Eatwell Plate. Use the Eatwell Plate to help you get the balance right. It shows how much of what you eat should come from each food group. Source: Public Health England.

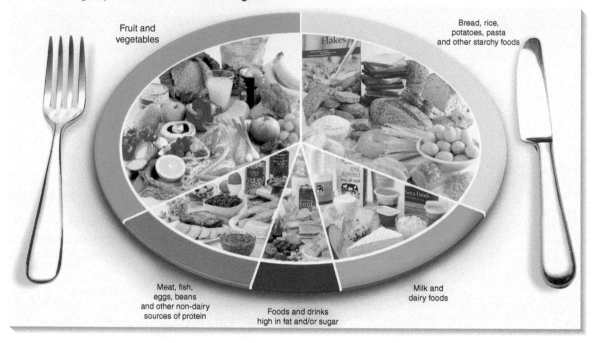

Fruit and vegetables

Bread, rice, potatoes, pasta and other starchy foods

Meat, fish, eggs, beans and other non-dairy sources of protein

Foods and drinks high in fat and/or sugar

Milk and dairy foods

Figure 43.2 Routes of enteral feeding.

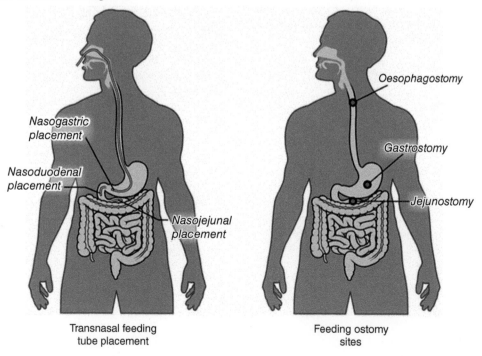

Nasogastric placement

Nasoduodenal placement

Nasojejunal placement

Oesophagostomy

Gastrostomy

Jejunostomy

Transnasal feeding tube placement

Feeding ostomy sites

District Nursing at a Glance, First Edition. Edited by Matthew Bradby.
© 2022 John Wiley & Sons Ltd. Published 2022 by John Wiley & Sons Ltd.

Human nutrition is the selection, preparation and ingestion of foods. For nutrition to be adequate, a person must receive certain essential nutrients that are vital to maintain health and wellbeing. They have a number of important functions: providing energy, building and maintaining body tissue and controlling metabolic processes such as growth and temperature regulation. Providing good nutritional advice and support to patients and their families is a key part of the community practitioner's role.

Balanced diet

A balanced diet provides the body with essential nutrition in the form of fluids, adequate essential amino acids from protein, essential fatty acids, vitamins, minerals and adequate calories. The requirements for a healthy diet can be met from a variety of plant-based and animal-based foods. A healthy diet supports energy needs without exposure to toxicity or weight gain from consuming excessive amounts. A properly balanced diet alongside exercise is important for lowering health risks, such as obesity, heart disease, type 2 diabetes, hypertension and cancer. The Eatwell Guide is a simple guide to healthier eating (NHS, 2019b). It highlights the different types of foods and the proportions they should be eaten in for a well-balanced and healthy diet (Figure 43.1).

Obesity

Obesity in the UK is increasing. In 2015, 58% of women and 68% of men were overweight or obese. No matter how healthy a person's diet is they can still be at risk of serious health problems if too much is eaten for their energy needs. Obesity is known to have adverse health-related complications such as an association with type 2 diabetes and coronary heart disease as well as increasing the risk of earlier death. Because of this, obesity costs the NHS billions of pounds in additional healthcare. Without action, obesity-related diseases will cost an extra £45.5 billion per year. In addition, the Covid-19 pandemic has demonstrated a strong association between obesity and disease mortality.

Undernutrition

Undernutrition occurs when people consume fewer daily nutrients than their body requires and can result in malnutrition. At any point in time it is estimated that more than 3 million individuals in the UK are at risk of developing malnutrition, with approximately 93% of those individuals living within the community in their own homes. It is suggested that 26% of patients receiving district nursing care are malnourished. The consequences of malnutrition include increased risk of mortality, impaired immune function, delayed wound healing, impaired respiratory and myocardial function, depression, apathy, fatigue and physical weakness.

Identification and screening

Community nurses and their colleagues play a vital role in the identification of nutritionally vulnerable individuals, screening for risk of malnutrition and obesity, and ensuring that timely, holistic and personalised interventions are implemented. Furthermore, there are many common nutritional and gastrointestinal disorders that can impact on a patient's nutritional status including dysphasia, gastroesophageal reflux disease, peptic ulcers and diverticular disease. Nutritional considerations are also important for patients with health conditions such as cardiovascular disease, renal and neurological disorders, diabetes, cancer and trauma.

Nutritional screening is a quick, simple procedure that should be undertaken by nurses and other healthcare professionals during the first meeting and at least within 24 hours of meeting the patient, as it is critical for the early identification of malnutrition or obesity. Community nurses who provide care for adults in their own homes are well placed to undertake screening for malnutrition in the primary care setting, because they generally visit patients regularly and undertake a holistic assessment.

Nutritional screening is not always carried out on a routine basis. This may be for several reasons including:

- Lack of support and organisational culture
- Time and resources to screen
- Acceptability of the screening tool
- Professional judgement as to what constitutes good nutritional screening
- The need for training and sharing good practice
- The need for enhanced communication.

Moreover, some patients may be less willing than others to comply with the procedure.

The best screening tools to consider using are those that have been rigorously tested and validated and are easy to use. The Malnutrition Universal Assessment Tool (MUST) is suggested as the 'gold standard' for use in all healthcare settings, including the community. However, like all nutritional screening tools, MUST has strengths and weakness and should be used critically. Body mass index (BMI) can be used to assess for both malnutrition and obesity, but the index is unable to distinguish between muscle and body fat and should not be used in isolation from other evidence. No single nutritional screening tool should be relied on for diverse populations and clinical areas and district nurses should be encouraged to test a variety of screening tools appropriate to the community setting.

Enteral feeding

Enteral feeding is used for malnourished patients or those at risk of malnutrition who have a functional gastrointestinal tract but are unable to maintain an adequate or safe oral intake. Percutaneous endoscopic gastrostomy (PEG) administration of enteral feeds is the most commonly used method of nutritional support for patients in the community. Patients in the community often perform the routine care of the PEG themselves, or with the help of their carer, supported by a multidisciplinary team consisting of GP, dietician and district nurse (Figure 43.2).

Kidney/renal health

44

Debbie Brown, QN

Figure 44.1   General anatomy of the human kidney.

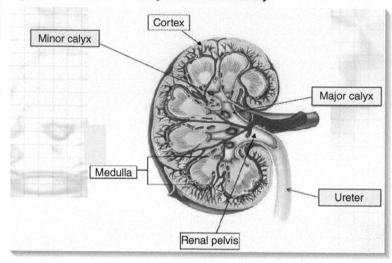

- Minor calyx
- Cortex
- Major calyx
- Ureter
- Medulla
- Renal pelvis

Figure 44.3   Glomerular capsule.

- Efferent arteriole
- Afferent arteriole
- Glomerular capsular space
- Parietal layer of glomerular capsule
- Proximal convoluted tubule
- Glomerular capillary covered by podocyte-containing visceral layer of glomerular capsule

Figure 44.2   Principal structure of the kidney.

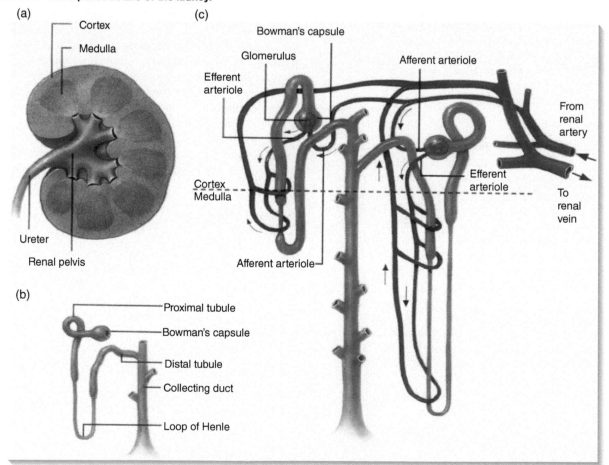

(a)
- Cortex
- Medulla
- Ureter
- Renal pelvis

(b)
- Proximal tubule
- Bowman's capsule
- Distal tubule
- Collecting duct
- Loop of Henle

(c)
- Bowman's capsule
- Glomerulus
- Efferent arteriole
- Afferent arteriole
- Efferent arteriole
- From renal artery
- To renal vein
- Cortex
- Medulla
- Afferent arteriole

District Nursing at a Glance, First Edition. Edited by Matthew Bradby.
© 2022 John Wiley & Sons Ltd. Published 2022 by John Wiley & Sons Ltd.

The kidneys are two bean-shaped organs, each about the size of a fist (Figure 44.1). They are located just below the ribcage, one on each side of the spine. Every day, the two kidneys filter about 180 litres of blood to produce about 2 litres of urine, composed of wastes and extra fluid. The urine flows from the kidneys to the bladder through two thin tubes of muscle called ureters.

Key anatomical points

Each kidney is made up of approximately one million filtering units called nephrons. The nephron includes a filter, called the glomerulus, and a tubule (Figure 44.2). The nephrons work through a two-step process. The glomerulus lets fluid and waste products pass through it; however, it prevents blood cells and large molecules, mostly proteins, from passing through.

The glomerulus (Figure 44.3) receives its blood supply from an afferent arteriole of the renal circulation. Unlike most other capillary beds, the glomerulus drains into an efferent arteriole rather than a venule. The resistance of these arterioles results in high pressure within the glomerulus, aiding the process of ultra-filtration, where fluids and soluble materials in the blood are forced out of the capillaries and into Bowman's capsule. Bowman's capsule is a cup-like sac at the beginning of the tubular component of a nephron that performs the first step in the filtration of blood to form urine.

The filtered fluid passes from the Bowman's capsule into the tubule, where needed minerals are reabsorbed back into the bloodstream and waste is removed as urine. Blood pressure is also autoregulated by the renal system and takes into account factors such as hydration, age, co-morbidities and medication. Together, this demonstrates how the kidneys are important because they keep the composition of blood stable by:

- preventing the build-up of wastes and extra fluid in the body;
- keeping levels of electrolytes, such as sodium, potassium and phosphate, stable as they are reabsorbed as needed;
- making hormones that help to:
  ○ regulate blood pressure,
  ○ make red blood cells,
  ○ support bone health.

Kidneys and ageing

As a person gets older, the kidneys have a decreased ability to eliminate toxins or prescribed drugs from the system. Therefore when treating older patients, be aware that some may need to have their dose reduced or medication stopped entirely. The rate at which the glomerulus itself filters blood should remain relatively constant; it is autoregulated based on factors such as hydration, medication, age and co-morbidities (e.g. diabetes or cardiovascular disease).

Community-specific considerations

The district nurse may be the first clinician to see the patient. The reason for the visit or requested task maybe to take routine bloods, assess a wound or administer an intramuscular or subcutaneous injection. This should also be an opportunity to check how the patient is feeling, for example to ask if they have noticed any changes or if they have any concerns.

Indications of kidney health can be seen in both the diagnostics of blood and urine samples and in the physical presentation of the patient. This may include the following:

- Hypertension
- Shortness of breath
- Bilateral lower leg/ankle oedema
- An increased need to urinate, particularly at night
- Itchy skin
- Muscle cramps
- Multisystem diseases with the potential to affect the kidney
- Family history of stage 5 chronic kidney disease.

Should a patient present with any of the above symptoms, a urine sample should be tested for protein by urine dipstick and also sent for ACR (albumin:creatinine ratio) test. This is a check for micro albuminuria, which should not be present in urine, as it is a larger molecule. If the test is positive, the test should be repeated with an early morning sample. If the ACR ratio is greater than 30 μg/mg, dip the sample for haematuria (blood in urine). This would indicate a need for referral to urology.

A blood test should be taken for urea and electrolytes, which will include the glomerular filtration rate; this is a marker of function of the kidneys. If there is a new finding of a reduced eGFR (estimated glomerular filtration rate), the test should be repeated within two weeks, to rule out acute kidney injury. Three samples over not less than 90 days are required to detect progression. From the age of 40, the kidneys can lose up to 1 milliliter of function per year.

If you notice any ankle or lower leg oedema, shortness of breath, an increased need to urinate or reduced urine output, this should alert to further investigation, starting by taking blood pressure (it is helpful to know the normal blood pressure for the patient). If the urinary volume is less than 0.5 ml/kg/hour for 6 hours in adults this could be an indication of acute kidney injury, which requires urgent management and should never be ignored. It is always advisable to contact the nurse in charge or the GP for further advice and support.

45 Skin assessment

Sandra Lawton, QN

Figure 45.1   Macules

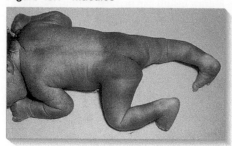

Figure 45.2   Papules

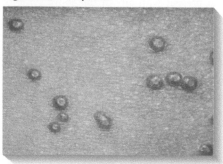

Figure 45.3   Plaques

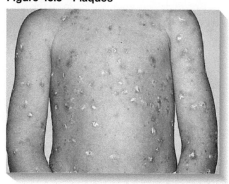

Figure 45.4   Wheals

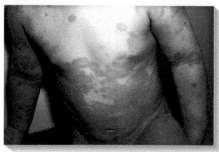

Figure 45.5   Vesicles

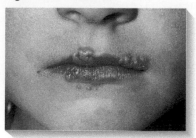

Figure 45.6   Pustules

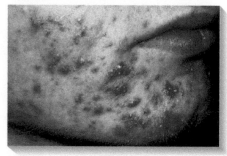

Figure 45.7   Crust

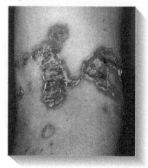

Figure 45.8   Lichenification.

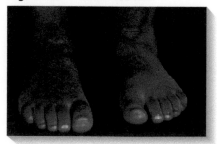

District Nursing at a Glance, First Edition. Edited by Matthew Bradby.
© 2022 John Wiley & Sons Ltd. Published 2022 by John Wiley & Sons Ltd.

Skin conditions are the most frequent reason for attendances in primary care. It is estimated that at any one time around 23–33% of people have a skin problem that can benefit from medical or nursing interventions. Surveys suggest around 54% of the UK population experience a skin condition in a given 12-month period, with most self-caring (69%) and around 14% seeking further medical advice, usually from a doctor or nurse in the community (Schofield et al., 2011).

Assessing a patient presenting with a rash

The skin should be examined in a warm, well-lit room, preferably with natural lighting or artificial lighting that will not change the natural skin colour.

Clinical history to be considered when examining a patient with a rash:

- Onset: acute or chronic?
- Systemic symptoms (fever)
- Duration of rash
- Change in rash over time: flare and remission
- Symptoms of rash (itching, pain, soreness)
- Family history of skin disease
- Recent contact with individuals with a rash (scabies, chickenpox)
- Drug history and medications
- Allergies
- Other medical history (atopy: asthma, hay fever)
- Does it occur at different times of the year?
- Do work/school/hobbies have an impact?
- Previous and present treatments and their effectiveness
- Are there any treatments, actions or behavioural changes that have influenced the condition?

Clinical examination

When examining the patient, use a gown or sheet to maintain dignity as each area of the skin is exposed for examination. Touching is an important aspect of the examination. It provides information about skin texture and temperature and also breaks down the physical barrier and stigma associated with skin disease. The skin should be examined thoroughly (from the scalp to toes including hair, nails and flexures), looking at the following features.

Distribution

Is the rash acral (hands, feet), in the extremities of ears and nose, in light exposed areas, or mainly confined to the trunk?

Shape

Are the lesions small, large, annular (ring shaped), or linear?

Skin types

With different skin colours and hair types, lesions, which in white skin appear red or brown, appear black or purple in skin of colour and mild degrees of redness (erythema) may be masked completely. Inflammation commonly leads to pigmentary changes – both lighter (post-inflammatory hypopigmentation) and darker (post-inflammatory hyperpigmentation), which may persist for a long time after the initial skin condition has settled.

Character

Is there redness (erythema), scaling, crusting, or exudate? Are there excoriations, blisters, erosions, pustules, papules? Are the lesions all the same (monomorphic, e.g. drug rash) or variable (polymorphic, e.g. chickenpox)? Lesions can further be defined as primary or secondary lesions.

Primary lesions

Primary lesions are present at the initial onset of the disease and include (Figures 45.1–45.6):

- *Macules* – a flat mark; circumscribed area of colour change: brown, red, white or tan.
- *Papules* – elevated 'spot'; palpable, firm, circumscribed lesion generally <5 mm in diameter.
- *Nodules* – elevated; firm; circumscribed; palpable; can involve all layers of the skin; >5 mm in diameter.
- *Plaques* – elevated, flat-topped, firm, rough, superficial papule >2 cm in diameter. Papules can coalesce to form plaques.
- *Wheals* – elevated, irregular-shaped area of cutaneous oedema; solid, transient, changing, variable diameter; red, pale pink or white in colour.
- *Vesicles* – elevated, circumscribed, superficial fluid-filled blister <5 mm in diameter.
- *Bulla* – vesicle >5 mm in diameter.
- *Pustules* – elevated, superficial, similar to vesicles but filled with pus.

Secondary lesions are the result of changes over time caused by disease progression, manipulation (scratching, rubbing and picking) or treatments. These include (Figures 45.7 and 45.8):

- *Scale* – heaped-up keratinised cells; flaky exfoliation, irregular, dry or oily, silver, white or tan in colour.
- *Crust* – dried serum, blood or purulent exudate; slightly elevated.
- *Excoriation* – loss of epidermis; linear area usually due to scratching.
- *Lichenification* – rough, thickened epidermis; accentuated skin markings caused by rubbing or scratching.

During clinical examination samples of scales, crusts, hair and nails may be taken. A skin biopsy may be appropriate with blistering rashes or when diagnosis is uncertain. Blood investigations may also be done, depending on diagnosis and assessment.

Coping with the skin condition

A great deal can be observed in the patient's expression and persona, which may give insight to how they feel and are coping with the skin condition. They may be withdrawn, not sleeping and be very conscious about their appearance and the reactions of others (staring, name calling or bullying. Within dermatology there are several psychological and disease-specific scores which can measure the impact of skin disease. For more information visit: https://www.cardiff.ac.uk/medicine/resources/quality-of-life-questionnaires

Further information is available from the British Dermatological Nursing Group (http://www.bdng.org.uk) and the Primary Care Dermatology Society (http://www.pcds.org.uk).

46 Continence

Debra Dooley, QN

Figure 46.1 Continence aids.

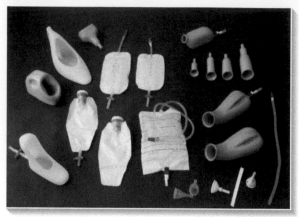

Figure 46.3 Anal irrigation kit. Source: Coloplast Corp.

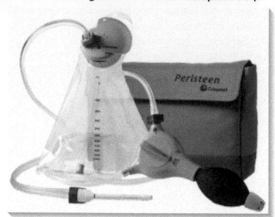

Figure 46.2 Anal plug. Source: Coloplast Corp.

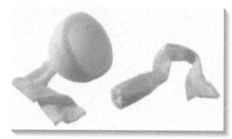

Figure 46.4 (a-e) Examples of proprietary incontinence products used in community healthcare.

(a)   (b)   (c)

(d)   (e)

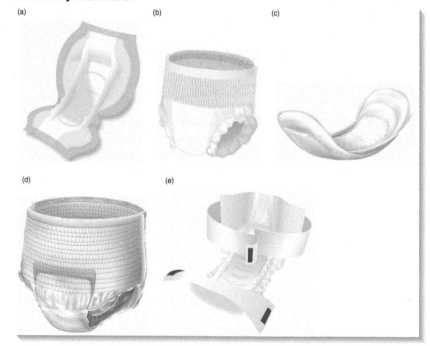

Incontinence is a symptom of an underlying medical disorder which results in the involuntary loss of urine or faeces and is neither gender nor age specific. It is a hidden disorder, not spoken about with family, friends or colleagues, and can affect confidence and dignity, leading to social isolation, breakdown in relationships, family stress and admission to residential care. In the UK, approximately 14 million people are affected by bladder dysfunction and 6.5 million with bowel dysfunction, more than the total suffering from diabetes, asthma and epilepsy combined. Rates for urinary incontinence are difficult to establish, due to the covert nature of the condition; however, best estimates are 1 in 4 females over 35 years of age and 1 in 10 adult males. Urinary and faecal incontinence affects 50–80% of care home residents. Financially, it has a vast impact on NHS expenditure. This is directly related to an ageing population, co-morbidities and inconsistency in the level of continence care provided across the UK.

Role of the district nurse

The role of the district nurse is often to listen, assess and signpost the patient to the most appropriate specialist service, namely the bladder and bowel services or continence service. An integrated continence service will offer specialist support, treatment and advice on all elements of bladder and bowel dysfunction, and they will develop robust clinical pathways into secondary care to ensure each patient is given the opportunity to achieve optimum outcomes. There are numerous innovative treatments, aids and adaptations that can cure, treat and effectively manage bladder and bowel dysfunction without resorting to a life of pad usage (Figure 46.1).

A sensitive and holistic continence assessment will include some or the following, dependent upon the competence of the nurse: onset, impact on quality of life, medical, surgical and obstetric history, and a medication review including over-the-counter remedies. The assessment will also look at lifestyle including weight, smoking and alcohol consumption. Furthermore, the patient's own coping and self-treatment strategies will be reviewed. Finally, the environmental factors including access to lavatory, social factors and the patient's motivation and goals, will be included.

Clinical assessment should include a minimum three-day frequency/volume chart and/or seven-day bowel chart and, if indicated, dietary chart. A review of types of fluid and volume intake, a pelvic floor muscle tone examination, urinalysis, abdominal palpation, digital rectal examination, bladder ultrasound and – if clinically indicated – flow rates and urodynamic investigations may be undertaken. These clinical investigations should only be performed by nurses with skills and knowledge of the anatomy and physiology of the bladder and bowel, its normal function and the ability to recognise abnormal function. The outcome of the assessment will result in a nurse diagnosis and initiation of conservative treatment options.

Diagnoses/types of incontinence

Stress urinary incontinence

Symptoms include urinary leakage on physical exertion, coughing and sneezing. Stress urinary incontinence (SUI) is associated with parity (the number of pregnancies carried), chronic constipation and obesity. Non-invasive treatment strategies include lifestyle modification, pelvic floor muscle exercises, biofeedback and vaginal cones. Minimal invasive treatment options include urethral bulking agents.

Overactive bladder

Overactive bladder affects approximately 12% of men and women. Symptoms may include urgency, with or without urge incontinence, frequency of micturition and nocturia. Treatment strategies may commence following exclusion of underlying pathology and infection. These include lifestyle modifications, reduction in caffeine intake (low acidic drinks), pelvic floor muscle exercises, behavioural modifications, bladder retraining and anti-muscarinic medication.

Neurogenic bladder

This may be caused by spinal cord injury, Parkinson's disease, cerebral vascular accident, dementia and multiple sclerosis. Symptoms include overflow, retention and urinary incontinence. Treatment depends upon the location of the injury and includes timed voiding, double voiding, prompted voiding, anti-muscarinics and clean intermittent self-catheterisation. There are also a number of surgical interventions available.

Functional incontinence and the frail elderly

This is associated with co-morbidities, including cognition, loss of muscle tone, lack of oestrogen, fear of falls, dizziness, constipation, urinary tract infection and polypharmacy including diuretics and opiates. Treatment options should be person specific and include lifestyle modification, medication review and rationalisation, environmental assessment with an occupational therapist and provision of appropriate aids and adaptations.

Faecal incontinence

Faecal incontinence is associated with childbirth, chronic constipation, anal sphincter damage, congenital conditions, rectal prolapse and diarrhoea. Symptoms include urgency of defaecation, incontinence and passive leakage of faeces. Treatment is dependent upon the cause and will include dietary modifications, lifestyle modification including weight management, adequate fluid intake, pelvic floor muscle exercises, anal sphincter muscle exercises, medication (e.g. titrating low-dose lopermide), anal plugs (Figure 46.2), transanal irrigation (Figure 46.3), environmental assessment to establish appropriate seating position and access to the lavatory and bowel habit training. Other secondary care options include percutaneous tibial nerve stimulation, sacral nerve neuromodulation and/or surgery (Figure 46.4).

Conclusion

Incontinence is a symptom of an underlying disorder, which can be readily treated, often cured, or at least managed effectively. It is vital that the clinicians undertaking these assessments are competent, motivated and able to diagnose and engage the patient or caregiver in the treatment. Conservative interventions have been demonstrated to cure the majority of incontinence. District nurses have a duty to signpost their patients to local continence services if active intervention is beyond their scope of competence. Robust clinical treatment pathways will drive the improvement and deliver improved quality of life, including a reduction in catheter-associated urinary tract infections, moisture lesions and pressure ulcers, which can be directly associated with poor continence care.

Constipation

47

Debbie Bromley, QN

Figure 47.1   The Bristol Stool Chart was developed by Dr. Ken Heaton at the University of Bristol and first published in the *Scandinavian Journal of Gastroenterology* in 1997. It remains in use as a tool to evaluate the effectiveness of treatments for constipation and as a clinical communication aid. Source: Lewis, S.J. and Heaton, K.W. (1997). Stool form scale as a useful guide to intestinal transit time. *Scandinavian Journal of Gastroenterology* 32: 920–924. Reproduced with permission of Taylor & Francis.

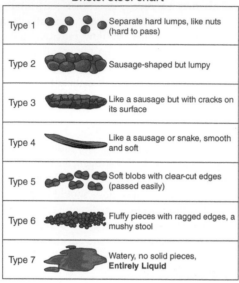

Bristol stool chart

Type 1	Separate hard lumps, like nuts (hard to pass)
Type 2	Sausage-shaped but lumpy
Type 3	Like a sausage but with cracks on its surface
Type 4	Like a sausage or snake, smooth and soft
Type 5	Soft blobs with clear-cut edges (passed easily)
Type 6	Fluffy pieces with ragged edges, a mushy stool
Type 7	Watery, no solid pieces, **Entirely Liquid**

Box 47.1   Some common symptoms of constipation.

- Abdominal bloating and excessive quantities of gas.
- Abdominal pain, often on lower left side, relieved by defecation or passing gas.
- Diarrhoea may be most severe on waking and may alternate with inconsistent constipation that may produce 'rabbit pellet' stools.
- Feeling that bowel is not completely empty.
- Mucus passing during defecation.
- Nausea and vomiting.
- Often full and not finishing meals.

Figure 47.2   Anatomy of the gastrointestinal tract. Source: rendixalextian/iStock/Getty Image.

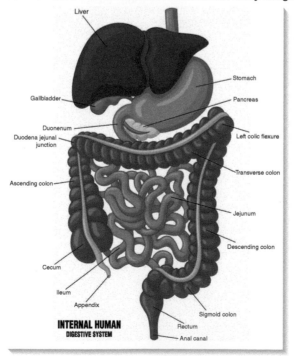

Constipation is defecation of infrequent hard/dry stools which may be difficult to pass and incomplete. Stools may be abnormally large or small and pellet-like, very dark in colour and often have an offensive odour. Large stools may be passed infrequently (e.g. every 3–10 days) or small stools may be passed daily. Chronic constipation can be identified when these symptoms have existed for longer than 8 weeks. Functional/primary/idiopathic constipation is constipation without a known cause. Secondary/organic is constipation caused by a medical condition or medication. Faecal impaction may occur with chronic constipation. The patient may present with acute abdominal pain, nausea, vomiting (faecal fluid in extreme cases), inability to pass a formed stool and 'overflow' of faecal fluid.

Prevalence

Constipation in the UK is variously estimated to affect between 8.2% and 52% of the population. This variation may be attributed to lack of definitive diagnosis and variable reporting/management by patients/healthcare professionals. It is known that twice as many women experience constipation as men and, whilst prevalent in all ages, the prevalence is greater in children, pregnant women, the elderly, and those with learning and physical disability. The condition may require years of management with pharmacology, diet, exercise and support.

Predisposing factors

Predisposing factors include poor dietary intake; lack of mobility; poor access/positioning on toilet; eating disorders; Hirschsprung's disease; anxiety; depression; pyrexia; dehydration; history of sexual abuse; diabetes mellitus; hypercalcaemia; hypokalaemia; hyperthyroidism; hypothyroidism; uraemia; autonomic neuropathy; cerebrovascular disease; multiple sclerosis; spinal cord injury/tumours; anal fissures/strictures; haemorrhoids; colonic strictures; inflammatory bowel disease; irritable bowel syndrome; obstructive lesions; rectal prolapse/rectocele; and post-natal/third-degree tears.

Medications which may cause constipation include antacids, antidepressants, anti-epileptics, antihistamines, antipsychotics, antispasmodics, antihypertensives, calcium supplements, diuretics, iron supplements and opioids.

Diagnosis

Diagnosis is based on assessment including history of predisposing factors and management to date; length of time the condition has existed; symptoms and size/frequency/colour/consistency/odour of stools (Box 47.1). Abdominal examination may be indicated but does not necessarily confirm/dispel a diagnosis of constipation. Use of the Bristol Stool Chart (Figure 47.1) can also support diagnosis and increase the patient's awareness, which can aid monitoring/effective management of the condition.

Complications

Complications include loss of sensory and motor function in the bowel, faecal incontinence, rectal bleeding, anal fissure, haemorrhoids, rectal prolapse, urinary tract infection, urinary incontinence, confusion, malaise, behavioural issues in children and young people, and loss of appetite/food refusal.

Management

Management should include effective treatment of any existing conditions (e.g. hypothyroidism, anxiety, dehydration) and management of predisposing factors (e.g. improved access to toileting facilities, exercise and dietary/fluid intake). The clinical research evidence indicates that management of diet/fluid intake alone is insufficient to achieve a good outcome for patients with chronic constipation. A patient-held diary may improve recording/communication and facilitate good management (Figure 47.2).

Medication

There are three groups of oral laxatives used to manage constipation. *Bulk-forming agents* include ispaghula husk, methylcellulose and sterculia. These should not be taken directly before bedtime and must be taken with an increased fluid intake. It takes 2–3 days for this group to be effective. Bulk-forming laxatives are not recommended in opioid-induced constipation, as their action is to distend the colon and stimulate peristalsis and opioids prevent the colon responding with propulsive action which may cause painful colic and sometimes obstruction. *Osmotic laxatives* work by retaining fluid in the gut and also take 2–3 days to be effective. Examples are lactulose and macrogols. *Stimulant laxatives* encourage the muscles in the gut to contract, making peristalsis more effective. They are designed to be used short term and work within 6–12 hours. Examples are senna, bisacodyl and sodium picosulphate. A stimulant laxative should be added if stools are soft but the patient finds them difficult to pass or complains of inadequate emptying. Faecal impaction may be treated in the first instance with bisocodyl suppositories or a docusate/sodium citrate enema. Paracetamol can be used to manage pain associated with constipation.

- A Cochrane review found sufficient evidence from 10 randomised controlled trials to conclude that of the osmotic laxatives macrogols are superior to lactulose in the management of chronic constipation (Lee-Robichaud et al., 2010).

There is general expert agreement in managing constipation: faecal impaction should be resolved before treating chronic constipation; a stepped approach to medication management including frequency and combination of laxatives should be employed. Regular reviews by a healthcare professional, adjusting the dose and combination of laxative therapy according to symptoms and promoting good diet/fluid/exercise routines may improve outcomes and recovery times.

Good clinical practice

The National Institute for Health and Care Excellence has produced six Quality Standard Statements for the management of children and young people with constipation (NICE, 2014). These highlight good clinical practice:

1 Full assessment
2 Oral macrogols as first-line treatment
3 Disimpaction treatment to be reviewed by a healthcare professional within one week
4 Maintenance therapy to reviewed by a healthcare professional within six weeks
5 Families receive written information regarding laxative management
6 If there is no response to treatment within three months patients are referred to a healthcare professional with expertise in the subject.

Catheter care

Debbie Myers, QN

Figure 48.1   A catheter. Source: Andrii Pohranychnyi/123 RF.

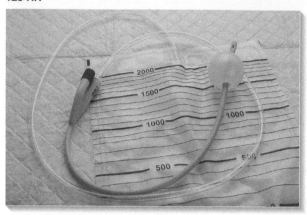

Figure 48.2   A drainage bag. Source: Sherry Yates Young/123 RF.

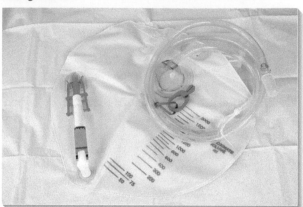

Figure 48.3   Emptying a drainage bag. Source: BSIP/Getty Images.

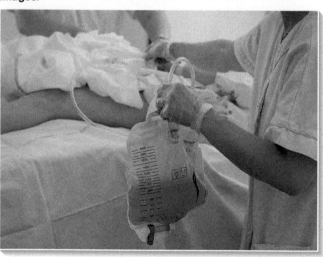

Figure 48.4   Tubing and bag secured to leg.

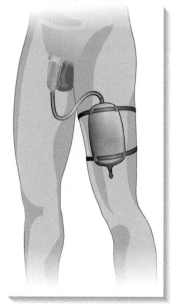

Strap the drainage
bag to the thigh

District Nursing at a Glance, First Edition. Edited by Matthew Bradby.
© 2022 John Wiley & Sons Ltd. Published 2022 by John Wiley & Sons Ltd.

All types of urinary catheterisation can be carried out in the community. Although common, urinary catheterisation is invasive and carries several risks including trauma and urinary tract infection (UTI). It should not be undertaken without full consideration of the risks, benefits and alternatives first. If catheterisation is required, intermittent catheterisation should be used in preference to indwelling catheterisation if appropriate and practical for the patient.

Assessment and documentation

A catheter may be inserted for the first time in the hospital or community. All patients should have a holistic assessment including:

- Reason for catheterisation
- Consideration of patient's/carer's ability to manage catheter
- Risk assessment (infection risk, confusion, environment, allergies).

    This assessment will help identify:

- Type of catheter to be used
- Lubrication
- Drainage system
- Suitable fixation devices.

    The ongoing need for an indwelling urinary catheter should be reviewed at each catheter change and a trial without catheter considered. Clinical reasons for continuing catheterisation should be documented. You must assess if the catheter is safe to be changed in the community by reviewing previous documentation or contacting the referrer if this information is not available.

Consent

Catheterisation is an invasive and intimate procedure and informed consent must be obtained following a discussion of the risks, benefits and ongoing management requirements. Consent must be obtained prior to the first catheterisation and at each subsequent catheter change. Where the patient is unable to give consent (e.g. unconscious or confused) a best interest decision can be made in line with the Mental Capacity Act and the rationale clearly documented.

    Catheters are available in a variety of materials, lengths and sizes (Figure 48.1).

Balloon inflation

The balloon should be inflated according to manufacturer's instructions. The balloon must never be topped up or deflated then re-inflated as this can distort the balloon and interfere with urine drainage or cause trauma to the urethra on removal.

Catheter insertion

Urinary catheterisation must be performed using an aseptic non-touch technique and aprons must be worn. An appropriate single-use lubricant should be used to aid urethral catheter insertion, as this reduces the risk of trauma and of infection (11 ml for male urethral and 6 ml for female urethral or suprapubic). The active ingredients in gels are different, so be aware of any sensitivities or contraindications (especially to lidocaine and chlorhexidine).

Drainage bags

Drainage bags are available in a range of sizes, tube lengths and tap styles. Selecting the right one for the patient will depend on a number of factors (Figure 48.2). Bags should be emptied when two-thirds full to prevent the weight pulling on the catheter, leading to trauma and risk of infection. Bags should be changed every 5–7 days and should not be disconnected for emptying or bathing. Overnight a night bag attached to the leg bag should be used for extra drainage capacity, removing the need for emptying overnight (Figure 48.3).

Fixation and support

Sleeves and straps are recommended to hold the leg bag and catheter in place (see Figure 48.4). This prevents tubing becoming trapped, leading to blockage or bypassing, and also prevents trauma or even erosion of the urethra due to traction on the catheter. Catheters and bags can be a source of pressure damage if not attached correctly, sat on or trapped.

Self-care

Routine catheter care should be performed by patients/carers to maximise independence and reduce infection risk. Advice, training and support must be given to allow them to do this safely.

Sex and catheters

People with catheters can continue a normal sexual relationship. Women can hold the catheter out of the way or tape it to their abdomen and men are advised to bend the catheter back along the length of their penis and cover it with a condom. In some cases patients may be taught how to remove and replace the catheter themselves to have sex, though this must be balanced with the risk of introducing infection. A suprapubic or intermittent catheter might be considered to be a suitable alternative.

Catheter-associated urinary tract infection

Patients with a catheter are at high risk of developing an infection and catheter-associated UTI (CA-UTI) can cause significant morbidity and sometimes mortality. Prior to handling the catheter/bags patients/their carers must always wash their hands with soap and water and carers must wear gloves.

    It is common for people with a catheter in for more than 90 days to have bacteria in their urine, therefore a CA-UTI is diagnosed in the presence of clinical symptoms of infection. If any of these symptoms are present the catheter must not be changed until antibiotic treatment has commenced. Those at high risk of developing a CA-UTI during routine catheter changes are usually prescribed prophylactic antibiotics to take prior to the catheter being changed.

Troubleshooting

If the catheter is bypassing/no drainage review the following:

- How much has the patient drunk? Could they be dehydrated? Is the urine concentrated?
- Is the tubing occluded, e.g. kinked or trapped between legs/in body folds or sat on?
- Is the drainage bag full and needs emptying?
- Is the drainage bag below the level of the bladder?
- Advise the patient to stand up and move around as this can promote drainage.

49

Recognising lymphoedema, lipoedema and chronic oedema in the community

Mary Warrilow, QN

Figure 49.1   Lipoedema.

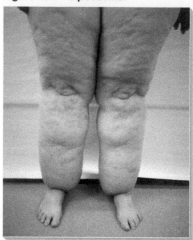

Figure 49.2   Severe bilateral leg Lymphoedema, showing skin folds and skin changes to the lower limbs.

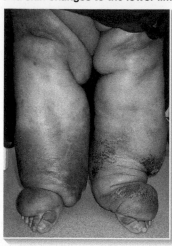

Figure 49.3   Secondary breast cancer related Lymphoedema.

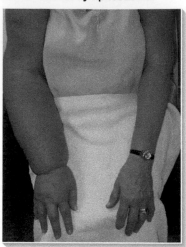

Figure 49.4   Hyperkeratosis and other skin changes are seen in chronic lymphoedema.

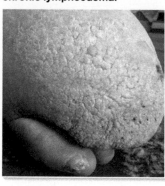

Figure 49.5   Dependent or gravitational oedema.

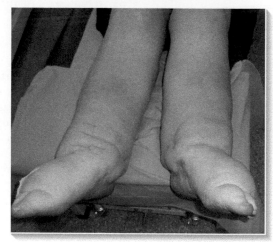

Figure 49.6   Multi-Layer compression bandaging treatment.

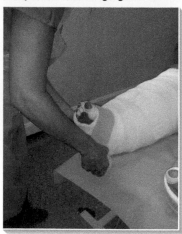

Table 49.1 Useful contacts and organisations.

British Lymphology Society	www.thebls.com
International Lymphoedema Framework	www.lympho.org
Lipoedema Ladies	www.lipoedemaladies.com
Lipoedema UK	www.lipoedema.co.uk
Lymphcare UK CIC	www.lymphcare.co.uk
Lymph-What-Oedema	https://lymph-what-oedema.com
Lymphoedema Support Network	www.lymphoedema.org

District Nursing at a Glance, First Edition. Edited by Matthew Bradby.
© 2022 John Wiley & Sons Ltd. Published 2022 by John Wiley & Sons Ltd.

The lymphatic system is sometimes a forgotten subject, with lymphoedema and lipoedema often being misunderstood and confused (Figures 49.1 and 49.2). The Lymphoedema Framework Project highlighted that lymphoedema is under-recognised and undertreated (Morgan et al., 2005) and similarly The UK Best Practice Guidelines for the treatment of Lipoedema (2017) also state that many with this condition are not recognised by healthcare professionals and misdiagnosed. However, awareness campaigns in recent years by patient and professional groups such as the Lymphoedema Support Group, Lipoedema UK and the British Lymphology Society have improved public and clinician awareness. Nurses have a duty to care, and greater awareness of the conditions and the importance of prompt referral and management are vital.

The lymphatic system

The lymphatic system is part of the immune system. It is a one-way drainage system composed of a network of initial lymphatic capillaries, deeper collecting vessels, lymph nodes and lymphatic organs such as the spleen and tonsils. The system returns excess interstitial fluid to the circulatory system and helps deal with bacteria, waste products and the absorption of fats from the digestive system. An impaired or damaged lymphatic system will result in impaired drainage and tissue swelling; this is lymphoedema.

Lymphoedema

Lymphoedema is a long-term condition (LTC) thought to affect more than 200,000 people in the UK. The condition is characterised by accumulation of fluid in interstitial places to cause swelling in the tissues in any part of the body but is commonly seen in the upper or lower limbs. The swelling can be classified as primary or secondary lymphoedema. Primary lymphoedema is genetic and due to malfunction of the lymphatic system. Secondary lymphoedema is due to damage to the lymphatic system, which can be as a result of cancer and its treatment, infection (cellulitis), trauma, and obesity. According to Cancer Research UK, breast cancer-related lymphoedema affects 1 in 5 women who have had breast cancer treatment (Figure 49.3).

Lymphoedema can have a huge impact on people's quality of life, affecting daily activities, mobility, and psychosocial morbidity. The symptoms include heaviness, aching and discomfort to the affected part of the body. There is also an increased risk of developing infection in the tissues (cellulitis) which could also lead to sepsis. This is due to the protein-rich lymph accumulation, which can encourage bacterial growth and a compromised immune system, due to failure in the lymphatic system. Chronic lymphoedema can lead to skin dryness, hyperkeratosis and papillomatosis (Figure 49.4).

Lipoedema

Lipoedema is characterised by accumulation and uneven distribution of adipose tissue, affecting the legs, hips and buttocks and sometimes the arms but with no swelling to the feet. Often a 'cuffing' effect is seen over the ankle. The skin is tender and bruises easily due to increased fragility of the capillaries. It almost exclusively affects women and is often mis-diagnosed as obesity or lymphoedema and is not well recognised by health professionals. Weight loss does not alter the lipoedema fat. The condition presents at puberty or at other hormonal fluctuations such as pregnancy or menopause.

As with lymphoedema, lipoedema can devastate both physical and mental health. pain, heaviness, fatigue and discomfort are common symptoms and the condition has a negative impact on an individual's quality of life.

Lipoedema UK recently undertook a survey of 933 women in the UK (Lipoedema UK 2021) as part of a response to The National Institute for Health and Care Excellence (NICE) new guidance on non-cosmetic liposuction in treating chronic lipoedema. The "Living with Lipoedema - non-cosmetic liposuction and other treatments" survey highlighted how the condition impacted on everyday life and that getting an early diagnosis was crucial in preventing progression. However, only 16% were diagnosed by their GP and 34% in a specialist clinic by a clinician or lymphoedema Nurse Specialist.

Chronic oedema

Chronic oedema can be caused by systemic failure (i.e. cardiac or renal failure, venous insufficiency and dependent oedema) (Figure 49.5). This type of oedema may lead to ulceration of the lower limbs.

Assessment, diagnosis and treatment

After referral, patients undergo a comprehensive holistic assessment, involving a full medical history including trauma, surgery, cancer/radiotherapy, the patient's lymphoedema/lipoedema history, and any previous treatments. Photographs, circumferential limb measurements and use of a moisture meter can be effective assessment tools. Assessment will also include examination of the swelling:

- Is the oedema pitting? Is the oedema in the arms or legs bilateral or unilateral? Does the patient bruise easily? Is there a family history of leg oedema?
- Are there any skin folds, thickening of the tissues, or skin changes?

This thorough assessment process will lead to a differential diagnosis and appropriate conservative or surgical treatment. Patients presenting with leg oedema/lipodema may require an arterial assessment to ensure that compression therapy in the form of bandaging, pneumatic compression therapy, or hosiery is not contraindicated. Referral for other investigations such as Fluoroscopy to track lymphatic vessels and pathways or scans to help with finding the cause of the lymphoedema can be very helpful.

Conservative Treatment for both conditions are similar.

Severe to moderate lymphoedema with a secondary lymphoedema will need an intensive phase of daily treatment over a 2–4 week period, known as decongestive lymphoedema treatment (Figure 49.6). This includes daily skincare, exercise and a combination of compression bandaging, specialist pneumatic compression therapy or medical lymphatic drainage to redirect lymph to areas that are not congested so fluid can drain normally.

The maintenance phase of treatment for lymphoedema/lipoedema can be managed effectively by life-long patient self-care, including skincare, exercise, simple lymphatic drainage and wearing appropriate compression garments. Patients will be monitored and reviewed during the maintenance phase and can be discharged from the lymphoedema service once stable. Other surgical interventions which are emerging include specialist non-cosmetic liposuction, lymph node transplant and lympho-venous anastomosis.

A placement with the local lymphoedema/lipoedema clinic is an interesting and rewarding experience that should inspire nurses to go on to develop their knowledge and raise awareness or even specialise in this area. Being able to recognise these conditions and refer on to a specialist team as necessary will ensure that patients receive appropriate care and treatment so that further complications and developing co-morbidities can be reduced or prevented.

A list of useful organisations are shown in Table 49.1.

50 Pressure ulcer prevention

Debbie Myers, QN and Neeshu Oozageer Gunowa, QN

Figure 50.1 Typical sites for pressure ulcers.

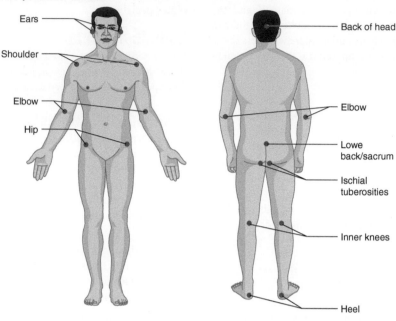

Ears
Shoulder
Elbow
Hip

Back of head
Elbow
Lowe back/sacrum
Ischial tuberosities
Inner knees
Heel

Figure 50.2 Risk factors.

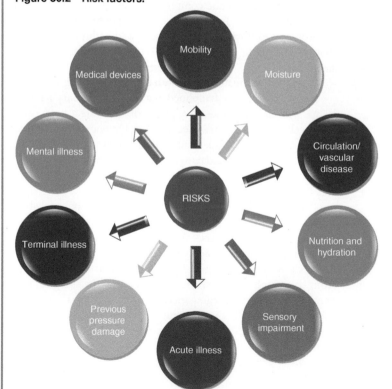

Mobility
Medical devices
Moisture
Mental illness
Circulation/ vascular disease
RISKS
Terminal illness
Nutrition and hydration
Previous pressure damage
Acute illness
Sensory impairment

Box 50.1 Associated assessments.

- Skin assessment
- Continence assessment
- Pain assessment
- Psychological assessment
- Assessment of mental capacity
- Moving and handling assessment
- Nutritional assessment
- Seating assessment

Box 50.2 Patient and carer education.

Education should cover:

- What a pressure ulcer is
- Why they form
- Where they form
- What to look for
- Preventative actions
- Positioning/repositioning advice (including frequency)
- How to use nay equipment provided including checking in working order
- Moving and handling techniques
- Skin inspection (including frequency)
- When and how to contact nursing team

Documentation should include:

- The education and advice given
- What the patient/carer has agreed to do
- The frequency of any interventions

District Nursing at a Glance, First Edition. Edited by Matthew Bradby.
© 2022 John Wiley & Sons Ltd. Published 2022 by John Wiley & Sons Ltd.

The European Pressure Ulcer Advisory Panel (EPUAP) defines a pressure ulcer as: 'A localised injury to the skin and/or underlying tissue usually over a bony prominence, as a result of pressure or pressure in combination with shear'. Figure 50.1 shows the most common locations for pressure ulcer development. They can occur in a patient of any age and can cause severe pain, harm or even death.

Risk factors

There are a number of factors that increase the risk of developing pressure ulcers (Figure 50.2). A holistic assessment is crucial to identify the risks and how to reduce them. Assessment should consider the following areas.

Mobility

- Can the patient mobilise/change position independently?
- If they need help, how often is this available?
- Is the patient bedbound or sitting for long periods in one position?
- Do moving and handling needs increase risk of friction and shearing forces?

Moisture

- Is the patient incontinent?
- Are any continence products used? Are they suitable for needs/changed at the frequency they need to be?
- Is the patient sweating?

Circulation/vascular disease

- Is the patient diabetic?
- Do they have any known circulatory problems?

Nutrition and hydration

- Is the patient over/underweight?
- Do they eat a well-balanced diet?

Sensory impairment

- Does the patient have normal sensory perception?
- If not, this poses a risk as normal perception of pain can stimulate movement and enable detection of pressure damage at an early stage.

Acute illness

- Is the patient acutely ill?
- This increases risk as it can affect mobility and nutritional intake.

Previous pressure damage

- Is there previous damage due to pressure?
- Skin remains vulnerable over site of previous damage so is at greater risk of breaking down.

Terminal illness

- Links with level of mobility, nutrition and circulation?
- Is the patient bed bound?
- Is the patient undergoing chemotherapy or radiotherapy?
- Is the patient taking steroids?
- Are body systems shutting down?

Mental illness

- Does the patient understand the risks and consequences?
- How motivated/able are they to manage risks?
- What is their ability to self-care?
- Is there a risk of self-neglect?

Medical devices

- Are medical devices causing increased pressure?
- A nasal cannula can cause pressure damage behind ears; a catheter can get trapped and cause pressure damage between the thighs.

Special considerations

- Although age itself is not a risk factor, the co-morbidities and frailty that often come with age may increase risk.
- Pain must be assessed as this may affect the patient's mobility and thereby contribute to risk of pressure damage. Consider if analgesia could be masking pain in pressure areas.
- Again not listed as a risk factor but important to consider is the increased risk people with darker skin tones are at developing more severe pressure ulcers due to delayed detection.

Many of these risk factors are linked, so a risk in one area presents a risk in another. It may be necessary to undertake more detailed risk assessments for some of these factors (Box 50.1) and referral to other services may be appropriate.

Interventions

Interventions to reduce the risk of pressure damage must be agreed with the patient and others involved in supporting them (formal and informal carers, care home staff). Plans must be individualised to the patient and their specific needs with training/education given as needed. It is important to document what advice and training has been given and what care has been delegated and to whom.

Interventions to reduce risks include:

- Advice and education related to risk factors (Box 50.2)
- Altering position (standing up; offloading)
- Provision of equipment – cushion; mattress; heel protectors. Can also use a cushion behind the back for those with a prominent spine
- Use of pillows (e.g. between knees; under calf with leg raised and foot overhanging edge to offload pressure on heels)
- Providing moving and handling equipment to prevent damage from friction and shearing forces if patient is moved inappropriately (e.g. hoist; slide sheets; turners).

A range of equipment made from different materials is available to cater for different levels of risk, though the specific equipment available will vary across organisations. Special equipment should not be used in isolation and it is not suitable in all cases. For example, heel protection may be needed through 'boots', but these may not be suitable for walking, so would present a risk in more mobile patients or those who are confused.

Concordance and safeguarding

Patients have the right to choose not to follow advice or use equipment provided, even when this may cause them harm. A nurse must be assured that a patient has made an informed choice based on understanding of risks and consequences. It may be beneficial to undertake an assessment under the Mental Capacity Act to ensure the patient has capacity to make this choice. If the patient lacks capacity, their carers must be involved in discussions though a nurse may need to make a decision in the patient's best interests and consider a safeguarding referral, if the carer is hindering effective care.

Where a patient is choosing not to follow advice/use equipment the nurse must make every effort to understand why. This will help determine if there is a suitable alternative even if that is not the most effective. For example, the patient may find a particular cushion uncomfortable but will accept an alternative. Always consider if there is a safeguarding concern and if in doubt speak to your safeguarding team. Causes for concern include potential self-neglect or carers not meeting the needs of the patient (e.g. repositioning; nutrition; toileting needs).

51 Lower leg ulceration

Carol Hedger, QN and Susan Knight, QN

Box 51.1   Types of leg ulceration.

- Venous leg ulcers – mainly due to chronic venous hypertension
- Arterial leg ulcers – caused by poor arterial blood supply
- Mixed leg ulceration – these have elements of both venous and arterial disease
- Other causes – sickle cell disease, Klippel–Trenauny syndrome, pyoderma gangrenosum, malignancy

Box 51.3   Signs and symptoms of venous and arterial ulceration.

Venous ulceration

- Pigmentation (brown staining) – caused by the breakdown of red blood cells trapped in the skin
- Induration (hard, woody feeling) – caused by fibrosis of the subcutaneous fatty layer, which can result in a champagne bottle-shaped leg
- Varicose eczema
- Atrophie blanche – areas or white skin stippled with red 'dots' of dilated capillary loops
- Oedema
- Ulcer above the ankle
- Ulcer over the malleolus

Arterial ulceration

- Dusky colour on foot/cold foot
- Loss of hair on the leg
- Atrophic shiny skin on the shin
- Thickened toe nails
- Loss of pedal pulses
- Ulcers on toes/heel/foot
- Pain the lower legs/foot when raised

Box 51.4   How to measure ankle–brachial pressure index (ABPI).

The patient should lie flat for at least 10–15 minutes, any restrictive clothing or bandaging/stockings should be removed.

Measuring the brachial pressure

1 Apply the correct-sized cuff around the upper arm and locate the brachial pulse; apply the correct ultrasound contact gel over the pulse
2 Place the Doppler probe at a 45 degree angle on the gel and move the probe to obtain the best signal
3 Inflate the cuff until the Doppler signal is lost then slowly deflate the cuff and record the pressure at which the signal returns
4 Repeat this procedure on the other arm
5 Use the higher of the two arm systolic pressures to calculate the ABPI

Measuring the ankle pressure

1 Apply the correct-sized cuff around the ankle immediately above the malleolus; protect any ulceration with cling film
2 Locate all the pulses on the foot (see Figure 51.1)
3 Apply the contact gel to the dorsalis pedis or anterior tibial pulse and apply pressure as described for the brachial pressure; record the result
4 Repeat this for either the posterior tibial or the peroneal pulses
5 Use the higher of the pulses in each foot to calculate the ABPI for each leg

For each leg: divide the higher ankle pressure (A) by the higher brachial pressure (B): A/B = ABPI.

Box 51.2   Risk factors for venous and arterial disease.

Venous disease

- Deep vein thrombosis (DVT)
- Thrombophlebitis
- Swollen legs
- Multiple pregnancies
- Past venous/orthopaedic surgery
- Varicose veins
- Previous leg ulceration

Arterial disease

- Ischaemic heart disease
- Hypertension
- Angina
- Diabetes mellitus
- Intermittent claudication
- Transient ischaemic attack (TIA)/stroke
- Myocardial infarction
- Rheumatoid arthritis

Figure 51.1   Location of foot pulses. Source: weerayut ranmai/123RF.

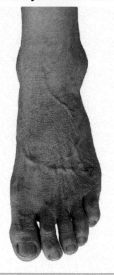

Box 51.5   Ankle–brachial pressure index (ABPI).

- >1.0 – intact arterial supply; consider full compression
- 0.8–0.9 – some arterial disease; consider full compression
- 0.6–0.8 – significant arterial disease; these patients may be suitable for reduced compression
- <0.5 – severe arterial disease; refer to a specialist nurse or vascular team
- >1.3 – suggestive of medial wall hardening; refer to specialist nurse or vascular team

District Nursing at a Glance, First Edition. Edited by Matthew Bradby.
© 2022 John Wiley & Sons Ltd. Published 2022 by John Wiley & Sons Ltd.

A venous leg ulcer is defined in the SIGN guidelines (www.sign.ac.uk) as an open lesion between the knee and the ankle joint that remains unhealed for at least four weeks and occurs in the presence of venous disease. A leg ulcer is not itself a disease but a manifestation of underlying problems. When assessing patients the healthcare professional must be aware that venous disease is not the only cause of lower leg ulceration (Box 51.1).

There a several reasons why patients develop lower leg ulceration. Nelzen (2008) highlighted that approximately 35% of cases have underlying co-morbidities, such as diabetes, lymphoedema and arthritis. As the age of the population increases so does the incidence. Guest et al. (2015) identified 730,000 patients with leg ulceration, equivalent to 1.5% of the adult population.

Anatomy and physiology

Venous leg ulcers occur because the valves connecting the superficial and deep veins are not working correctly. This reduces venous return and can lead to congestion and ankle oedema. The veins contain small fragile valves which help prevent back flow of blood. These are easily damaged by thrombosis, or can simply not close properly if the patient stands for long periods – as the action of walking assists with the return of venous blood when the calf muscle exerts pressure – or is pregnant or obese.

The oedema causes capillary pressure to increase and blood cells can leak through the porous capillary walls into the surrounding tissue as the congestion increases. The mechanical pressure exerted by the tissue oedema and trapped cells causes stretching of the skin and the vessels in the microcirculation. This is believed to cause tissue damage, which will lead to ulceration or poor wound healing, especially following trauma to the lower leg.

Patients with peripheral vascular disease (PVD) are more likely to have arterial ulceration, mainly caused by impaired circulation as a result of narrowing of the arteries. This can be caused by atherosclerosis, making the vessels less elastic and less responsive to the pumping action of the heart. Diabetic patients are at risk of peripheral neuropathy and PVD, leading to the development of neuro-ischaemic or ischaemic ulceration. It should be noted that any ulceration on the foot of a diabetic patient should be reviewed as diabetic foot ulceration and not lower leg ulceration.

Presentation and assessment

Sometimes patients present with slow-to-heal leg wounds that they have attempted to manage themselves; during patient assessment many will cite trauma, for example insect bites or a knock, as the initial cause of the damage. It is important to investigate the patient further for underlying circulatory problems and associated co-morbidities to explain why their injury has failed to heal. The assessment must be holistic and should include screening the patient's past medical history for risk factors (Box 51.2)

and examining the patient for classic signs and symptoms of venous and/or arterial disease (Box 51.3).

Arterial status should be investigated by Doppler ultrasound assessment (Box 51.4) using a hand-held Doppler. The Doppler uses an ultrasound signal to capture the movement of red blood cells as the pressure is released from the sphygmomanometer cuff applied sequentially to the arms and legs. The readings obtained during the assessment are used to calculate the ankle–brachial pressure index (ABPI), which is the ratio of blood pressure in the lower legs to the blood pressure in the arms. The ABPI provides an indication of possible arterial occlusion in the lower leg (Box 51.5). The Doppler assessment of ABPI should not be taken in isolation but used as part of the whole assessment to determine the correct diagnosis and treatment for the patient.

Management of leg ulceration

Following holistic assessment and discussion with the patient to develop a care plan, treatment should start as soon as possible. If assessment indicates that the patient is suitable for compression, the choice will depend on the experience and competency of the healthcare professional, the extent of the tissue damage and patient preference.

Best practice would support the application of compression bandaging, but this requires an appropriate level of knowledge and skill and should not be undertaken by someone without training, as poorly applied compression bandaging can result in damage or may act as a tourniquet when the bandages slip down. If the level of lower leg oedema is not excessive and the limb is of normal size and shape, then consideration can be given to the application of compression stockings. Several manufacturers produce two-layer leg ulcer management kits. These include a low compression dressing retention sock, which is applied immediately over the dressing and a second (usually open toe) compression sock. The level of compression supplied with these kits is generally between 35 and 40 mmHg at the ankle. It is important to measure the patient's limb accurately to ensure that the correct level of compression is supplied.

Conclusion

The early implementation of appropriate evidence-based assessment and treatment of patients with lower leg wounds can reduce healing times considerably. Delay in assessing patients can lead to further complications such as repeated cellulitis, chronic oedema/lymphoedema of the lower leg leading to increased patient distress, pressure on nursing services and financial burden to the NHS. Managing patients with leg ulceration can be a complex challenge for any healthcare professional, even the most experienced.

Further information can be found at SIGN (Scottish Intercollegiate Guidelines Network) https://www.sign.ac.uk/

52 Management of type 2 diabetes in the older person: using the International Diabetes Federation Guidelines in practice

Sonia Wijesundera, QN, Julie Phipps, QN, and Marion Snelling, QN

Box 52.1   Comprehensive geriatric assessment for older people with diabetes.

A. Microvascular complications
- Retinopathy: Screening for diabetes retinopathy and other ocular diseases common in older people (cataract, glaucoma and macular degeneration)
- Preservation of vision to prevent social isolation, reduce incidence of falls and maintain independence especially for self-administration of insulin
- Nephropathy: Chronic kidney disease is common in older age. Monitoring of renal function is essential for adjustment of medications. Angiotensin-converting enzyme inhibitors or angiotensin receptor blockers should be used in patients with persistent microalbuminurea
- Neuropathy: Regular inspection of feet and access to diabetes foot care is essential in older people with diabetes, as many may not be able to care for their feet due to physical disability

B. Cardiovascular risk factors
- Cardiovascular disease is the most common cause of mortality in patients with diabetes regardless of age. Lifestyle modifications such as weight reduction, regular physical activity.and smoking cessation is recommended. Achieving blood pressure and blood glucose control is essential along with dyslipidaemia treatment and the use of antiplatelets as a secondary prevention

C. Geriatric syndromes: screening for the following geriatric syndromes should be addressed in the initial assessment
- Cognition: Cognitive impairment should be suspected if difficulties in self-care develop.
- Physical function: Mobility, gait, balance and ability to perform activities of daily living
- Nutrition: Oral health, chewing, swallowing and hydration
- Depression: Suspect if non-concordance with medication develops
- Co-morbidity burden
- Polypharmacy: Medication review to reduce medication burden
- Pain: Assessment for neuropathic or non-neuropathic pain
- Urinary incontinence: This could be the first manifestation of diabetes
- Social status: The need for help in self-care, especially for those on insulin

Source: Abdelhafiz, A.H. and Sinclair, A.J. (2013). Management of type 2 diabetes in older people. *Diabetes Therapy* 4(1): 13–26. Licenced under CC BY 2.0.

Figure 52.1   Withdrawing medication from a vial.

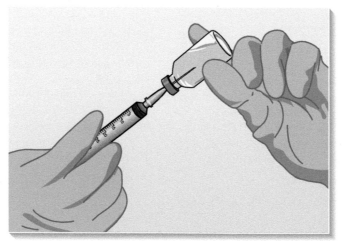

Diabetes mellitus is a group of metabolic diseases characterised by hyperglycaemia resulting from defects in insulin secretion, insulin action or both. There are two main types of diabetes:

- Type 1 diabetes, accounting for about 10% of diabetes diagnosis, results from autoimmune destruction of pancreatic beta cells, which leads to absolute insulin deficiency.
- Type 2 diabetes, accounting for 90% of diabetes incidences, is characterised by a decline in beta cell function and worsening of insulin resistance.

Type 2 diabetes is more prevalent in middle-aged or older people, due to impaired pancreatic islet cell function and increased insulin resistance. It is also three times more common in people of African and Afro-Caribbean origin. The cost of direct patient care for those living with type 2 diabetes in the UK was estimated at £10 billion in 2017 (Diabetes UK, 2017) and prescribing for diabetes accounts for around 10% of the total cost of prescribing in England and Wales. With a rising ageing population, the diagnosis and cost of type 2 diabetes is predicted to increase.

Challenges when caring for an elderly person with type 2 diabetes

The aim of registered nurses working with any patient is to promote health, prevent illness and alleviate suffering. Nurses could face a number of challenges when they provide care for an older person with type 2 diabetes, such as coexisting medical conditions, cognitive and physical dysfunction and polypharmacy. Furthermore, recurrent hospital admissions due to infection, hyper- and hypoglycaemia and falls are common among this group (Box 52.1).

Care planning

Care planning for the older person with type 2 diabetes is often challenging (Figure 52.1). Complications of type 2 diabetes and ageing can affect the individual's learning capabilities, ability to self-care, functional status, maintaining safety and independence. The common geriatric syndromes that nurses may come across and require assessment include:

- Falls
- Pain
- Urinary tract infection
- Cognitive impairment
- Depression
- Hypoglycaemia
- Polypharmacy
- Delirium.

Hypoglycaemia in the older person with type 2 diabetes is common if they are treated with glucose-lowering medication. This is associated with declining renal and liver function and nutritional deficits. Furthermore, in type 2 diabetes the levels of counter-regulatory hormones, such as glucagon, decline, contributing to predominance of neuroglycopenic symptoms. Hypoglycaemia in the older person can increase the risk of falls, affect memory and lead to hospital admissions. Repeated hypoglycaemia episodes can cause emotional distress to the person even if they are mild episodes.

In 2013, the International Diabetes Federation (IDF) published guidelines for the management of type 2 diabetes in older people. The guidelines are useful to understand how the management of diabetes is closely associated with factors such as functional status, presence of frailty and dependency, co-morbidity profiles and life expectancy of the older person. The guidelines enable clinicians who work with older people to incorporate a number of assessments into a management tool defined as the comprehensive geriatric assessment (CGA). The CGA is then linked with advice on safe glucose-lowering therapies, prevention of hypoglycaemia, main aspects of patient safety, avoiding unnecessary hospital admissions and aged care home residency.

The management of hyperglycaemia in the older person with type 2 diabetes is another example where the IDF guidelines can be applied to develop a care plan. It is essential that hyperglycaemia in the older person is managed according to functional status. The HbA1c target between 53 and 59 mmol/mol is appropriate for a functionally independent older person, whereas for a functionally dependent person with frailty it can be between 53 and 64 mmol/mol. It is important to reduce hyperglycaemia symptoms (tiredness, polyuria and polydipsia) and dehydration, which are associated with hyperglycaemic hyperosmolar status and ketoacidosis.

Self-management of type 2 diabetes

Educating the older person with type 2 diabetes and the family/carer about both hypo- and hyperglycaemia prevention and management should be included in the care plan. This will enable them to recognise and treat hypo- and hyperglycaemia effectively within their own care setting, and understand when the person requires immediate medical attention.

Physical and cognitive dysfunction in older type 2 diabetics can have a significant impact on diabetes self-management as well as quality of life. It is recommended that a comprehensive geriatric assessment should be carried out in addition to the diabetes assessment in order to find out the best approach to manage their diabetes.

Nurses working with older persons with type 2 diabetes have a key role to ensure that a comprehensive initial assessment is performed to enable effective care planning. The IDF guidance is a valuable tool that supports nurses to ensure that the functional status, comprehensive clinical monitoring, medication-related issues, cognitive and mental health, pain, and falls risk are all included in the assessment to plan type 2 diabetes care for the older person.

53 Ischaemic heart disease

Lynne Bax, QN and Helena Masters, QN

Figure 53.1   Ischaemic heart disease.

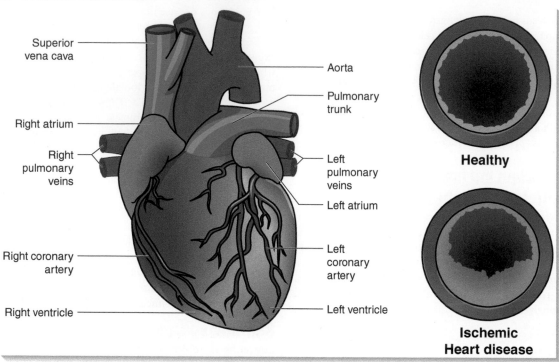

- Superior vena cava
- Aorta
- Pulmonary trunk
- Right atrium
- Right pulmonary veins
- Left pulmonary veins
- Left atrium
- Right coronary artery
- Left coronary artery
- Right ventricle
- Left ventricle

Healthy

Ischemic Heart disease

Figure 53.2   A human blood vessel.

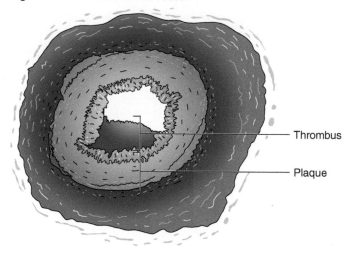

- Thrombus
- Plaque

Figure 53.3   A Holter monitor applied to male patient. Source: rumruay/Shutterstock.

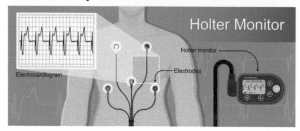

Holter Monitor

Electrocardiogram

Holter monitor

Electrodes

District Nursing at a Glance, First Edition. Edited by Matthew Bradby.
© 2022 John Wiley & Sons Ltd. Published 2022 by John Wiley & Sons Ltd.

What is ischaemic (or coronary) heart disease?

Ischaemic heart disease is a condition characterised by reduced blood supply to the heart, the term 'ischaemic' meaning 'a reduced blood supply'. The heart is supplied with blood via the coronary arteries, so a blockage in these blood vessels will be responsible for a reduced blood supply to the heart muscle in ischaemic heart disease. It can also be referred to as coronary artery disease and is the most common cause of death in most Western countries. Reduced blood supply to the heart results in a reduced oxygen supply to the muscle and can ultimately lead to heart attack (Figure 53.1).

Causes

Most ischaemic heart disease is caused by atherosclerosis. This is a chronic condition where over time atherosclerotic plaques build up in the bifurcations of major arteries in the body, such as the coronary arteries. The buildup of plaque can result in an obstruction of the lumen of the coronary arteries over time, reducing the passage of blood through to the heart muscle. Ischaemic heart disease can also be the result of a sudden severe narrowing or closure of the large coronary artery or the coronary artery end branches when the covering of an atherosclerotic plaque ruptures, allowing debris to be passed into the bloodstream (Figure 53.2). This can in turn lead to a heart attack, although heart attacks caused by artery narrowing alone are rare.

Ischaemia is most likely to occur when the heart demands extra oxygen, such as during exertion (activity), eating, excitement or stress, or exposure to cold. Coronary artery disease can progress to a point where ischaemia occurs even at rest.

Ischaemia, and even a heart attack, can occur without any warning signs and is called 'silent' ischaemia. Silent ischaemia can occur in anyone with heart disease, though it is more common among people with diabetes.

Two tests are used to diagnose ischaemia: the exercise stress test and the Holter monitor – a battery-operated portable device that measures and records the patient's electrocardiogram (ECG) continuously, usually for 24–48 hours (Figure 53.3). Other tests also may be used.

When ischaemia is relieved in less than 10 minutes with rest or medications, it is known as 'stable coronary artery disease' or 'stable angina'.

Risk factors for atherosclerosis

Atherosclerosis can be caused by lifestyle habits and other conditions, such as:

- Smoking
- Hypertension (high blood pressure)
- High cholesterol level
- Lack of regular exercise
- Being obese or overweight.
- Having a family history of coronary heart disease (CHD). The risk is increased if you have a male relative with CHD under the age of 55 or a female relative under 65
- Diabetes.

Symptoms

The most common symptom of coronary artery disease is angina (also called angina pectoris). Angina is often referred to as chest pain. It is also described as chest discomfort, heaviness, tightness, pressure, aching, burning, numbness, fullness or squeezing. It can be mistaken for indigestion or heartburn. Angina is usually felt in the chest, but may also be felt in the left shoulder, arms, neck, back or jaw.

Other symptoms that may occur with coronary artery disease include:

- Shortness of breath
- Palpitations (irregular heartbeats, skipped beats or a 'flip-flop' feeling in your chest)
- A faster heartbeat
- Dizziness
- Nausea
- Extreme weakness
- Sweating.

Treatment

Treatments for CHD include lifestyle changes, medicines and medical procedures. Treatment goals may include:

- Relieving symptoms
- Reducing risk factors in an effort to slow, stop, or reverse the buildup of plaque
- Lowering the risk of blood clots forming - particularly focused on efforts to stop plaques rupturing as platelets often aggregate to form a thrombus at the site of rupture. Fragments of the clot can break away and can cause an embolism in other vessel beds which can then also lead to heart attack
- Widening or bypassing clogged arteries.

Preventing complications of coronary heart disease

In order to achieve these treatment goals there are various treatment options, including:

- Coronary interventions, such as angioplasty and coronary stent
- Coronary artery bypass grafting (CABG)
- Medications – organic nitrates, beta blockers, calcium channel blockers, statins and aspirin.

Tips for district nurses on assessment of patient

- Identify how much knowledge of disease process the patient has
- Has the patient been referred to cardiac rehabilitation, if appropriate?
- Is a specialist nurse input needed?
- Are they on the correct medications according to the national guidelines?
- Are they concordant with their medication?
- Does the patient understand their risk factors?

Respiratory health

Dorothy Wood, QN, Mags Dowie, QN, and Lee Hough, QN

Figure 54.1   Sources of indoor pollutants.

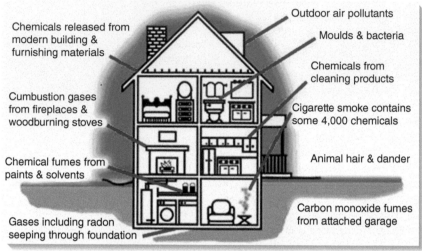

Chemicals released from modern building & furnishing materials

Cumbustion gases from fireplaces & woodburning stoves

Chemical fumes from paints & solvents

Gases including radon seeping through foundation

Outdoor air pollutants

Moulds & bacteria

Chemicals from cleaning products

Cigarette smoke contains some 4,000 chemicals

Animal hair & dander

Carbon monoxide fumes from attached garage

Table 54.1 BODE (BMI, airflow obstruction, dyspnoea and exercise capacity) parameters.

	Points				
	1	2	3	4	Score
Body mass index data measured using the BMI measuring device	<21	≥21			
Airway obstruction data measured in FEV$_1$ using the airway obstruction measuring device	>65%	54–64%	36–49%	≤35%	
Respiration rate data measured in breaths/min using the respiration rate sensor	14–17	18–21	22–25	>25	
Physical activity data (distance in meters) measured using the activity monitor	≥350	250–349	150–249	≤149	
				Total	

Factors affecting respiratory health

The risk factors affecting chronic respiratory and pulmonary diseases (CRD) have been well documented, but by far the worst risk factor is smoking. Future studies are also expected to show that Covid-19 symptoms are worse for smokers. Major respiratory risk factors include:

- *Tobacco smoke*: Both active and second-hand exposure to tobacco smoke is a major threat to people in all walks of life. It contains thousands of chemicals, 250 of which are known to be carcinogenic. The cumulative effect of tobacco smoke is known to contribute to irreversible obstructive changes in the lungs and increases the risk of CRD. Exposure to tobacco smoke is the leading cause of chronic obstructive pulmonary disease (COPD), and known to increase the incidence of childhood asthma, and the risk of childhood respiratory problems, lung cancer and cardiovascular disease. The source of most second-hand smoke is cigarettes and other tobacco products.
- *Indoor air pollutants* including solid fuels have been associated with asthma and COPD. The main indoor pollutants are tobacco smoke, allergens, carbon monoxide, mould, household products, and building materials such as asbestos and lead (Figure 54.1).
- *Outdoor air pollutants*: Long-term exposure to traffic-related air pollution may shorten life expectancy and is a risk factor for cardiac, pulmonary and lung cancer mortality. However, the impact of outdoor air pollution appears to be smaller than that of cigarette smoke.
- *Occupational agents*: In 2000 the World Health Organization estimated that risk factors in the workplace were responsible for 13% of COPD, 11% of asthma and 9% of lung cancers worldwide.

Improving respiratory health

Respiratory diseases are often complex with multiple phenotypes. Exposure to pollutants contributes to disease progression and increases the risk of acute exacerbations. Reducing exposure to these pollutants is clearly a big step to improving respiratory health. In addition to being the leading cause of COPD, continued exposure to tobacco smoke will result in increased neutrophilic inflammation in COPD patients. In asthmatic patients, continued exposure to smoke may result in steroid resistant asthma, resulting in patients having poor control of their condition. Ultimately, increasing damage leads to increasing breathlessness so smoking cessation is clearly an important aspect of promoting lung health.

Identification of occupational exposure to pollutants which triggers respiratory symptoms should be encouraged. Occupational lung disease remains one of the most common work-related injuries: injury to lung tissue results from inhalation of air contaminants. Although silicosis may be on the decline, hypersensitivity pneumonitis is now recognised as an occupational disease resulting from exposure to allergens.

Viral infection can impair host defences and increase the risk of secondary infection and colonisation with pathogenic bacteria.

Annual flu vaccination has the potential to reduce patient morbidity, mortality and unplanned hospital admission and should be strongly encouraged. If a patient has more than two chest infections annually, refer on for investigations to rule out potential co-morbidities such as lung cancer, bronchiectasis or TB.

Pulmonary rehabilitation is the most effective non-pharmacological means of reducing breathlessness by using exercise and education to reverse the effects of deconditioning and can reduce mortality risk in COPD. COPD does not have to be a progressive disease if the patient keeps fit and stops smoking.

Systemic inflammation contributes to significant morbidity, in particular metabolic abnormalities, weight loss, muscle weakness and wasting, cardiovascular disease, depression, osteoporosis, cancer and anaemia. Being aware of the multisystem effect of respiratory disease will ensure you provide appropriate advice and support.

Management of respiratory health

The management of various respiratory conditions depends on the age of the patient and also the severity of the disorder. Managing the patient's condition, symptoms and their own expectations is usually a multifactorial and shared approach between healthcare practitioner, patient, family and carers. A child with asthma may require instructions on how and when to use inhalers, and the child's parents may need informing of severe warning signs and general health promotion. An adult with a chronic long-term lung disease such as COPD will need advice on smoking, dust, weather changes and remaining as active as possible, as well as regular check-ups and monitoring of medications and lung function.

The general care of a patient with a lung condition includes various management options including smoking cessation, medications and inhalers (short-acting, long-acting, steroids, secretion-reducing medications, nebulisers, oxygen), regular reviews including spirometry and peak flow measurements, care plans, emergency rescue medications (antibiotics and steroids) and rehabilitation (Table 54.1). The most important management interventions are stopping smoking (if a smoker) and maintaining lung health by limiting infections and improving general wellbeing.

Care plans for patients with respiratory conditions are vital to maintaining health and preventing possible rapid decline. Studies have shown that regular reviews and reaffirming plans with patients can reduce the progression and exacerbations of the condition, and result in increased adherence. Ideally, goals should be set and evaluated at each review to individualise and centre the care on the patient's needs.

Managing exacerbations and infections should be planned for beforehand between the nurse and patient/carers. Worsening symptoms, infections, exacerbations and red flag warning signs should be discussed. Often care plans include signs and symptoms of worsening episodes, what to do when, and who to contact.

55 Chronic obstructive pulmonary disease

Lynne Bax, QN and Helena Masters, QN

Figure 55.1   Symptoms of COPD.

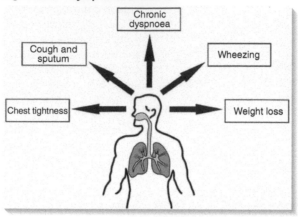

Chronic dyspnoea

Cough and sputum

Wheezing

Chest tightness

Weight loss

Figure 55.2   Medical interventions for COPD: bronchodilators. Source: Prime Medic Inc.

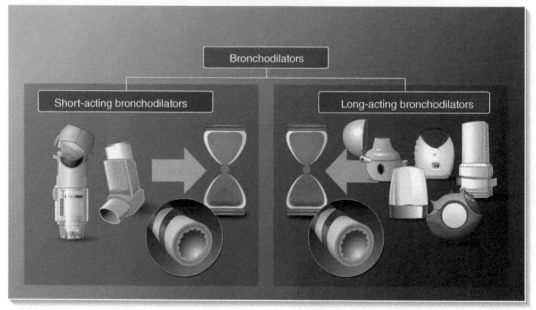

Bronchodilators

Short-acting bronchodilators

Long-acting bronchodilators

Figure 55.3   A nurse offers one-to-one support. Source: Marjorie Johnson.

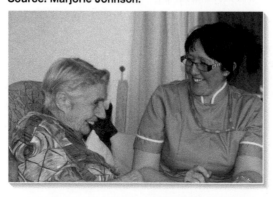

Figure 55.4   Supporting a patient with inhaled therapy.

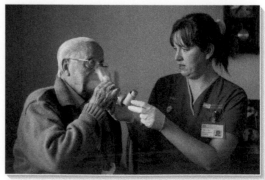

District Nursing at a Glance, First Edition. Edited by Matthew Bradby.
© 2022 John Wiley & Sons Ltd. Published 2022 by John Wiley & Sons Ltd.

What is COPD?

Chronic obstructive pulmonary disease (COPD) is a condition that affects the airways of the lungs. It is characterised by airflow obstruction that is not fully reversible. This obstruction is usually progressive in the long term and is often referred to as a long-term condition. COPD is predominantly caused by smoking, however other factors, particularly occupational exposures, may also contribute to its development.

Symptoms

Symptoms may include the following (Figure 55.1):

- Chronic cough
- Breathlessness on exertion
- Regular sputum production
- Frequent winter 'bronchitis'
- Wheeze.

Diagnosis

A diagnosis of COPD should be considered in patients over the age of 35 years who present with symptoms. Diagnosis occurs through clinical presentation, physical examination and confirmation using spirometry. The National Institute of Health and Care Excellence (NICE, 2018) defines COPD as airflow obstruction with a reduction in forced expiratory volume in one second and forced vital capacity (FEV_1/FVC ratio), such that FEV_1/FVC is less than 0.7. In addition to this, the Medical Research Council (MRC) dyspnoea scale can be used to grade breathlessness, a typical symptom of COPD, according to the level of exertion required to provoke it.

COPD exacerbations

An exacerbation of COPD is defined as a sustained worsening of the patient's symptoms from their usual stable state which is beyond normal day-to-day variations, and is acute in onset. Exacerbations occur often with commonly reported symptoms being worsening breathlessness, cough, increased sputum production and change in sputum colour.

Managing exacerbations

The frequency of exacerbations can be reduced by appropriate use of inhaled corticosteroids, bronchodilators, antibiotics and vaccinations (NICE, 2018). Important issues for community nurses to consider for managing exacerbations are:

- Supporting patients in self-management on responding promptly to the symptoms of an exacerbation
- Starting treatment with oral steroids and/or antibiotics
- Referring patients for non-invasive ventilation when indicated
- Supporting patients with hospital-at-home or virtual ward schemes.

Treatments

Self-management

A major problem associated with COPD is the occurrence of exacerbations and the periodic worsening of symptoms. The concept of self-management is to teach and educate patients to effectively manage their symptoms and condition, including the unscheduled use of antibiotics and oral corticosteroids taken for symptom relief in an exacerbation (Rennard and Calverley, 2003). NICE (2018) supports the use of self-management guidance which encourages patients to respond promptly to the symptoms of an exacerbation, and requests that patients should be given rescue medication (antibiotics and oral corticosteroids that are reserved for use in a serious attack or exacerbation of COPD) to keep at home for use as part of their self-management strategy (Figure 55.2).

Stopping smoking

It is important to encourage and support all patients with COPD who are current smokers to stop smoking, regardless of the stage of their COPD. Stopping smoking can help to reduce the frequency of exacerbations (Figure 55.3).

Inhaled therapy

Although there is no cure for COPD, inhaled medications can help. They can improve symptoms and a person's quality of life. Inhaled medicine can be with an inhaler or a nebuliser. There are different types of inhalers available and it is important that patients are taught the correct way to use their inhaler to get the most benefit from their inhaled medicines (Figure 55.4).

Pulmonary rehabilitation

Pulmonary rehabilitation is an exercise and education programme for patients with COPD. It should be made available to all appropriate people with COPD including those who have had a recent hospitalisation for an acute exacerbation. Studies show that patients who attend pulmonary rehabilitation programmes have better outcomes in terms of exacerbations and disease progression.

Use non-invasive ventilation

Non-invasive ventilation is a treatment option for patients who suffer from hypercapnic ventilatory failure during exacerbations, and who do not respond to usual inhaled and oral therapy. It is usually provided within a hospital environment by specially trained staff.

Nutrition

It is important that patients with COPD have a healthy, well-balanced diet that contains all food groups. Patients with COPD require more energy for breathing compared to people without COPD and this puts them at risk of significant weight loss, which can result in muscle wastage. In order to maintain their weight in a normal range, patients need to increase their energy intake through a varied and energy-rich diet. The evidence also suggests that a poor diet may be linked to increased infections (exacerbation). It is also advisable for patients with COPD to drink plenty of non-caffeinated drinks. Increasing fluid intake helps to keep the mucus produced by the lungs thin; this will make coughing up this mucus easier (expectorating).

Rest

It is important for patients with COPD to get adequate rest and conserve energy. There are many ways to conserve energy and these include planning activities ahead to allow for rest periods, getting a good night's sleep, and not planning activities for directly after a meal. They should also avoid overstretching themselves on days when they are not feeling at their best.

56 End-stage respiratory care in the community

Jenny Rasmussen, QN

Figure 56.1 Lung function and disease trajectory in cancer and COPD.

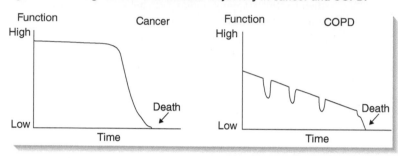

Table 56.1 Symptoms reported in the last 12 months of life.

Symptoms	COPD	Lung cancer
Dyspnoea	76%	60%
Pain	56%	56%
Cough	46%	40%
Nausea/vomiting	39%	45%
Anorexia	15%	19%
Constipation	65%	55%

Figure 56.2   NICE summary of holistic care and pathways that patients with end-stage respiratory disease should be offered, with a multidisciplinary approach adopted.

Step 1	Step 2	Step 3	Step 4	Step 5	Step 6
Discussions as the end of life approaches	Assessment, care planning and review	Coordination of care	Delivery of high quality services in different settings	Care in the last days of life	Care after death
• Open, honest communication • Identifying triggers for discussion	• Agreed care plan and regular review of needs and preferences • Assessing needs of carers	• Strategic coordination • Coordination of individual patient care • Rapid response services	• High quality care provision in all settings • Acute hospitals, community, care homes, hospices, community hospitals, prisons, secure hospitals and hostels • Ambulance services	• Identification of the dying phase • Review of needs and preferences for place of death • Support for both patient and carer • Recognition of wishes regarding resuscitation and organ donation	• Recognition that end of life care does not stop at the point of death. • Timely verification and certification of death or referral to coroner • Care and support of carer and family, including emotional and practical Bereavement support

Social care

Spiritual care services

Support for carers and families

Information for patients and carers

District Nursing at a Glance, First Edition. Edited by Matthew Bradby.

In the UK, over half of respiratory deaths are caused by lung cancer and chronic obstructive pulmonary disease (COPD). However, people with end-stage respiratory disease are often unprepared for the progressive nature of their disease and are dying without discussing palliative care options or advanced care plans.

One of the challenges around this is that end-stage respiratory diseases are often very unpredictable. In COPD, the disease trajectory is typically a slow decline with an increase in frequency of acute exacerbations that sometimes end in unexpected death. Patients with interstitial lung disease (ILD) have a more predictable deterioration, with an increased dependence on oxygen following episodes of hypoxia and respiratory failure. End-of-life care starts at diagnosis for some people with ILD who have rapidly progressing illness or advanced disease at the time of diagnosis. See Figure 56.1 for disease trajectory comparisons.

Clinical indicators of advanced lung disease

- Cachexia: low body mass index (<21)
- Increased hospital admissions for infections or respiratory failure
- Severe airways obstruction (FEV_1 <30%)
- Severe restrictive disease (vital capacity <60%, transfer factor <40%)
- Meets criteria for long-term oxygen therapy (LTOT): persistent hypoxia (PaO_2 <7.3 kPa)
- Persistent, severe symptoms despite optimal tolerated treatment
- Breathlessness limiting daily activities between exacerbations, at rest or on minimal exertion
- Symptomatic right-side heart failure
- Combinations of other factors, e.g. anorexia, depression, previous ITU admissions or need for non-invasive ventilation.

Once these patients are recognised they should be discussed regularly at palliative care meetings within practice, so that those who are approaching the end of life are offered full assessments. They should have the opportunity to discuss their needs and preferences for current and future treatment and to develop an advanced care plan detailing these preferences.

Why do patients with end stage disease suffer from uncontrolled symptoms?

Death normally occurs after a prolonged functional decline associated with a heavy symptom load. Over 75% of these patients are breathless in the last year of life, and in nearly half of these, the breathlessness is unrelieved by treatment. Breathlessness resulting from ILD is usually associated with hypoxia, unlike in COPD, where it is usually a combination of deranged airflow dynamics and air trapping. Common symptoms in the last 12 months of life as listed in Table 56.1. Psychological morbidity is also high with almost 90% having clinically relevant anxiety and depression.

Treatment of symptoms

During end-stage respiratory disease, healthcare professions must offer patients holistic, multidisciplinary care pathways (Figure 56.2). Some healthcare professionals may be hesitant about proactively managing symptoms due to concerns about the adverse effects of some pharmacological interventions, such as respiratory depression from opioids and anxiolytics. The main treatment for COPD is bronchodilators.

In ILD, oxygen is often used when oxygen saturations drop below 92% at rest. Often small increases in mobility cause a desaturation in this client group and this should also be assessed. In patients with chronic hypoxaemia, long-term oxygen therapy (LTOT) should be prescribed after appropriate assessment when the (arterial oxygen) PaO_2 is consistently at or below 7.3 kPa when breathing air during a period of clinical stability. These assessments are carried out by specialists and referral to them should be made promptly after two separate episodes of clinically stable oxygen saturations <92%.

Clinical stability is defined as the absence of exacerbation of chronic lung disease for the previous 5–6 weeks, which often difficult to achieve. In addition, LTOT can be prescribed in chronic hypoxaemia patients when the clinically stable PaO_2 is between 7.3 kPa and 8 kPa, together with the presence of one of the following:

- Secondary polycythaemia
- Clinical and or echocardiographic evidence of pulmonary hypertension.

The oxygen flow rate must be sufficient to raise the waking oxygen tension above 8 kPa (60 mmHg). Once started, this therapy is likely to be life-long. LTOT is given for at least 15 hours daily. This includes night time because of the presence of worsening arterial hypoxaemia during sleep. This protects organs from the effects of hypoxia, which shortens life and is not prescribed for breathlessness although patients often perceive an improvement.

Short burst oxygen therapy refers to the intermittent use of supplemental oxygen at home, usually for periods of about 10–20 minutes at a time to relieve dyspnoea. Despite extensive prescriptions of short burst therapy, there is no adequate evidence available for firm recommendations and further research is required. The provision of oxygen will not be of clinical benefit to patients with normal saturations and alternatives should be explored, such as:

- A cool air fan and an open window
- A cold flannel or cold water spray
- Physiotherapy – breathing exercises
- Cognitive behavioural therapy and pacing of activities
- Relaxation techniques
- Making sure the inhaler technique are optimised (use of spacer).

Other drugs commonly used for both breathlessness and anxiety

Lorazepam (0.5 µg–2 mg) is a good anxiolytic and given submucosally, so absorbs quickly and is often used instead of diazepam, which, although longer acting, can cause longer episodes of drowsiness. Once the patient is more unwell midazolam via a syringe driver can be given. Oral morphine (2.5 mg four times daily) is effective for dyspnoea relief and pain relief. Its side effect of constipation should be anticipated. This dose can be titrated under supervision.

Neurological conditions

57

Victoria Queen, QN

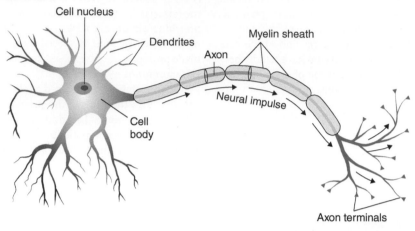

Figure 57.1   A human Neurone.

Cell nucleus

Dendrites

Axon

Myelin sheath

Neural impulse

Cell body

Axon terminals

Figure 57.2   Acute spinal injury.

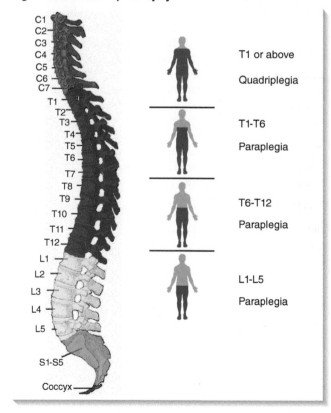

C1
C2
C3
C4
C5
C6
C7
T1
T2
T3
T4
T5
T6
T7
T8
T9
T10
T11
T12
L1
L2
L3
L4
L5
S1-S5
Coccyx

T1 or above

Quadriplegia

T1-T6

Paraplegia

T6-T12

Paraplegia

L1-L5

Paraplegia

Figure 57.3   Supporting and assessing a patient with paralysis.

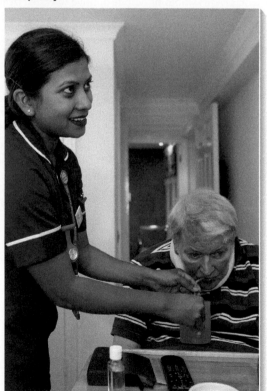

There are many different types of neurological conditions, which result from damage to the spinal column, brain or nerves. This damage is normally caused by illness or injury but many causes still remain unknown. Research is continuously being undertaken to understand why individuals develop certain neurological conditions, such as multiple sclerosis and Parkinson's disease (Figure 57.1).

Some neurological conditions are life-long and people can experience them at any point, such as those due to traumatic brain injury, whereas others are present from birth. The appearance of different neurological disorders can vary within a lifetime, for example muscular dystrophy commonly appears in early childhood, but Alzheimer's disease and Parkinson's disease (PD) generally affect mature adults.

Progression can also vary greatly, with some people who have experienced a stroke, for example, showing areas of improvement over time. In contrast, neurodegenerative conditions, such as multiple sclerosis and motor neurone disease (MND), will cause deterioration over time, affecting a person's quality of life and independence. Some neurological conditions, such as a brain tumour, are life threatening whereas some forms of Parkinson's disease, for example, have shown little impact upon life expectancy.

Some of the most common neurological conditions and their impact upon individuals, families, and carers are described in this chapter.

Paralysis

Paralysis is a common neurological condition. It is defined as the loss of the ability to move one or more muscles, and it can also cause loss of feeling and some bodily functions. Paralysis is normally caused by spinal nerve damage, head injury or stroke. It can be localised if a specific body part is paralysed, such as one hand, or generalised. Generalised paralysis affects larger body areas such as below the waist (paraplegia). Terms used to describe the location of paralysis include tetraplegia, also known as quadriplegia, where both arms and both legs are paralysed (Figure 57.2).

There are specialist centres across the UK providing rehabilitation for people with paralysis such as that from spinal injury. The impact of paralysis upon individuals and their families can be significant, however many people with paralysis lead fulfilling and successful lives.

Motor neurone disease

MND is a rare condition, but one that may require the support of community nurses. It is a progressive damage to the nervous system, causing severe muscle weakness and wastage, resulting from neurone cell death in the brain and spinal cord. Motor neurones control essential muscle activity, including walking, swallowing and gripping. Because MND is a progressive condition, some or all activities of daily living will become difficult or impossible with time. The exact cause of most MND is still poorly understood: there is a strain of hereditary MND but this only accounts for around 5% of cases.

In the early stages of MND individuals may experience a weakened grip, which can cause difficulty picking up or holding objects, drop foot or slurred speech. As the disease progresses, individuals may require support with all activities of daily living, for example with communication and mobility.

Parkinson's disease

PD is one of the most common neurological conditions in the UK. It is an umbrella term for a multitude of possible symptoms which result from cell death in an area of the brain called the substantia nigra. These can include, but are not limited to: tremor, bradykinesia (slowness of movement) and rigidity (muscle stiffness). The onset of PD can vary but commonly affects people over the age of 65. PD is complex to diagnose and requires a medical specialist to perform diagnosis. Progression of the disease is variable, with some forms developing very slowly over many years and others, such as those linked to head injury, progressing very quickly.

New treatments for the symptoms of PD are being developed continuously and at this point in time treatment of symptoms by medication has the best impact to enable people with PD to remain independent. Medication can be in the form of tablets, patches, injections, infusions or via gastrostomy. Brian surgery can also be an option for certain types of PD or for people with certain types of tremor.

Role of the district nurse

The district nurse has an important role in supporting people with neurological conditions, improving the quality of life and aiding independence. District nurses can provide support and nursing interventions in people's own homes, to enable them to remain independent (Figure 57.3). This may include, but not be limited to, supporting a person with PD to inject themselves with apomorphine, or a dopamine agonist that can be used as treatment for the symptoms of PD. District nurses can also support individuals to provide their own bladder and bowel care in paralysis, as well as signposting patients and their families to local support groups. There is a wide network of charities across the UK running branches and support groups. In addition they often support research regarding cures and treatments.

Multiple sclerosis

58

Julie Matthews, QN and Kathy Franklin, QN

Figure 58.1   Diagram of the human body showing those parts of the anatomy affected by Multiple Sclerosis. Source: VectorMine/Adobe Stock Photos.

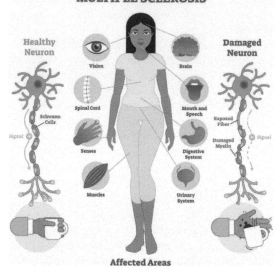

MULTIPLE SCLEROSIS

Healthy Neuron — Vision — Brain — Damaged Neuron — Schwann Cells — Spinal Cord — Mouth and Speech — Exposed Fiber — Signal — Senses — Digestive System — Damaged Myelin — Signal — Muscles — Urinary System

Affected Areas

Table 58.1 Management of multiple sclerosis.

Site of damage	Likely symptom
Spinal cord	Spasticity, weakness
	Bladder issues, bowel problems
Brainstem	Double vision and nystagmus
Optic nerve	Optic neuritis
Cerebellum	Balance, coordination, vertigo and tremor
Areas involved in thoughts and emotions	Cognition and depression
Symptoms not identified in any specific area	Speech and swallowing, fatigue and pain

Table 58.2 Health professionals involved in supporting people with multiple sclerosis.

Neurologist		GP	OT
DM therapy clinic	↔	↔	Physiotherapist
Neurorehabilitation		MS	Continence nurse
Urologist	↔	↔	SALT
Ophthalmologist		Specialist	Adult social services
Pain clinic	↔	↔	Dietician
Psychiatrist		Nurse	Podiatrist
Psychologist			

DM, Disease modifying therapy; SALT, speech and language therapy.

Multiple sclerosis (MS) is the most common neurological disease in young adults, particularly among Northern Europeans. It is a disease of the central nervous system (CNS) and involves the brain, spinal cord and nerves of the eye. It is thought to be an autoimmune disease in which the immune system attacks myelin surrounding the nerve fibre, causing inflammation, demyelination and interruption to nerve signals. It is estimated that approximately 100,000 people are affected by this disease in the UK. Currently, there is no cure for this condition.

Diagnosis

About 85% of people with MS are diagnosed with the type that manifests in a series of relapses (sometimes called an attack or exacerbation) followed by periods of good or complete recovery (a remission). About 75% of people whose disease pattern begins with relapsing and remitting symptoms later develop secondary progressive MS which, as its description suggests, denotes continuous deterioration. Unfortunately, 10–15% of people with MS are diagnosed with a form of the disease in which disability increases from the point of diagnosis. This is known as primary progressive MS.

Diagnosis usually involves a combination of investigations and many of the symptoms that people present with are not unique to MS. The evidence to make a diagnosis requires the use of magnetic resonance imaging (MRI) to identify two or more areas of scarring in different parts of the CNS that have occurred at different points in time. These are known as the McDonald criteria.

Symptoms

The effect that MS has on an individual depends on where the damage has occurred in the CNS and which nerve pathways are interrupted or blocked. Although the complexity of the CNS and how it manages information is still not fully understood, certain areas are associated with specific functions that ultimately produce specific symptoms. Figure 58.1 and Table 58.1 help to identify the site of damage and the symptoms that may be experienced.

Treatment and therapies

The basis of MS management has been and continues to be the management of symptoms with the goal of improved quality of life. There are now a number of disease-modifying therapies that are licensed for relapsing remitting MS. However, as our understanding of MS improves, we know that relatively simple things that people with MS can implement for themselves increases the likelihood that their symptoms can be controlled. Eating healthy foods, exercising regularly, keeping a 'steady' lifestyle and maintaining social activities are all helpful in this respect.

Under the NHS Constitution (England), every person has the right to be involved in discussions about their healthcare and be given information to enable them to do so. The National Service Framework for Long Term Conditions (Department of Health and Social Care, 2005) states that people with long-term neurological conditions are to have the information they need to make informed decisions about their care and treatment and, where appropriate, to support them to manage their condition themselves.

The majority of people with MS are fairly active and employed in a variety of occupations in the early years. For those that have had the condition for 15–20 years, more care provision may be needed, depending on their specific disabilities.

Living with the complex needs of a person who has MS can bring challenges for everyone involved, including carers and family. It is essential that everyone involved has the support they need and that a complete care package is provided by the various services available. Such a care package should address physical needs, psychological issues, including practical help and financial requirements.

It is essential that a care plan is formulated at the earliest opportunity so that individual care can be identified, planned and implemented. Holistic assessment identifies physical, emotional, social and spiritual needs, preferences or challenges. These are likely to change as various needs arise.

Whatever decisions people with more severe MS and their families decide to make, it helps if health and social care is coordinated by a multidisciplinary team. The involvement of different professionals should ensure that complex symptoms associated with severe MS are managed appropriately; together they can work towards preventing additional complications and ultimately hospital admission. MS specialist nurses may be available to help coordinate community-based services. These may include district nurses, health visitors, community matrons, neurophysiotherapists, community occupational therapists and adult care managers. GPs can refer patients to the neurologist and MS service and provide regular health monitoring. Table 58.2 helps to explain the pivotal role that an MS nurse can provide.

Palliative care provision should be available for all patients with life-limiting illnesses, regardless of diagnosis and should not be restricted to the last few days, weeks or months of life. The nursing input needed to help people manage MS will inevitably change over time.

Cancer as a chronic condition

59

Ben Bowers, QN

Figure 59.1 Time since diagnosis in people with cancer between 1991 and 2010, UK. Source: Modified from *The Rich Picture: People with Cancer*. Macmillan Cancer Support 2015.

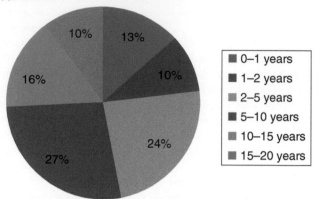

- 0–1 years
- 1–2 years
- 2–5 years
- 5–10 years
- 10–15 years
- 15–20 years

Figure 59.2 District Nurse administering chemotherapy in the home.

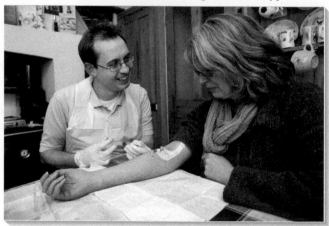

Box 59.1 Local cancer support services to consider.

- Maggie's Centers (based in certain hospitals but offer open access to a wide range of support, advice and groups to anyone living with cancer and their family and friends). https://www.maggiescentres.org
- Macmillan Cancer Support (the national website has a lot of useful advice and information. There is a link to local services supported by the charity). http://www.macmillan.org.uk/in-your-area/choose-location.html. National advice number: 0808 808 00 00
- Specialist Nurses caring for people with specific cancers are a great resource for advice on the type of local support groups that are running and which ones might be the most suitable for the individuals needs
- Cancer-site specific charities (national charities often have local support groups or online communities where people can access peer support and advice). Examples include:
  - Breast Cancer Care: https://www.breastcancercare.org.uk/in-your-area/support-events. Support line 0808 800 6000
  - Prostate Cancer UK: http://prostatecanceruk.org/get-support. Support line 0800 074 8383
- Oncology treatment centres have local cancer support groups and carer support groups advertised in their waiting areas.
- Local hospices are increasingly running support groups for people living with life-limiting conditions but not at the end of their lives.
- Citizens Advice (can offer financial advice and information or ways can access government benefits and voluntary services support). https://www.citizensadvice.org.uk

Box 59.2 Common long-term and late effects of cancer and its treatment.

Physical effects
- Memory problems
- Persistent hair loss
- Nausea and vomiting
- Fatigue
- Pain
- Altered nerve sensations
- Heart disease
- Lymphoedema
- Sexual difficulties
- Osteoporosis
- Dry mouth/altered taste
- Urinary problems
- Bowel problems

Psychosocial effects
- Mental health problems
- Body image issues
- Fatigue
- Sexual problems
- Financial difficulties
- Reduced confidence

District Nursing at a Glance, First Edition. Edited by Matthew Bradby.
© 2022 John Wiley & Sons Ltd. Published 2022 by John Wiley & Sons Ltd.

About 2.5 million people in the UK were estimated to be living with cancer in 2015. With advances in treatment, more than half of this population has been living at least 5 years after diagnosis and a quarter beyond 10 years (Figure 59.1). The focus of care is increasingly shifting to support people not just through initial treatment but also in living with and surviving cancer.

Having cancer and treatment can have lasting physical and emotional effects for the individual and their family. Relationships can change and ongoing symptoms can impact on social activities and work. Some people adjust constructively, drawing strength and new meaning from their experiences. However, a quarter of people report facing poor health after treatment. Depending on the cancer, some people may be having long-term cancer treatment in the form of chemotherapy or hormone therapies.

Holistic assessment

No two people living with cancer have the same needs and priorities. Healthcare services have traditionally focused resources on managing physical cancer treatment symptoms but now need to adapt to provide tailored individualised cancer survivorship and supportive care. District nurses often have contact with patients having ongoing cancer treatment or living with cancer as a chronic or palliative condition. Being aware of the long-term effects of cancer and treatments can help district nurses anticipate and meet needs.

There is a national drive for patients completing active treatment to receive a treatment summary detailing potential side effects, symptoms and consequences to watch out for. This should be sent to their GP to help inform future care. Not all patients and their GPs receive this written information as yet but it is becoming standard practice. It is worth sourcing this information to back up conversations and to help with empowering patients to self-manage and access suitable advice if they get new symptoms.

District nurses are well placed to make a holistic assessment, support self-management, and link individuals to appropriate support. Enabling individuals and their families to talk openly about their experiences can uncover a myriad of issues and worries that may go unnoted by medical colleagues. Actively listening to concerns and knowing what cancer support services exist locally (Box 59.1) is helpful in empowering individuals to access extra help to manage their symptoms and concerns.

Late effects of treatment

All cancer treatments impact on healthy body tissue in some way and can have different consequences. These consequences may happen straight away and lessen with time or may be long term and more constant. Some effects may even only emerge months after completing treatment. Box 59.2 highlights the most prevalent long-term and late effects of cancer and its treatment.

Each treatment has different potential long-term effects depending on the drugs used and what part of the body is targeted.

For example, some chemotherapy drugs can lead to nerve damage, osteoporosis or cataracts. Radiotherapy to the pelvic area can cause skin changes, infertility, lymphoedema, urinary and bowel problems. Long-term hormone therapies can cause memory problems, hot flushes, osteoporosis and weight gain. Regardless of treatment, it is common to experience ongoing fatigue.

Most people can be supported to effectively self-manage and lessen the long-term effects of treatment. Key to this is supplying suitable tailored information and signposting individuals to the right support. Rather than assuming that a symptom cannot be lessened or resolved, it is important to help the individual access the right care. Macmillan Cancer Support, Cancer Research UK and cancer disease site-specific charities have very informative patient information on symptoms and what may help. Local oncology services and palliative care services often have access to specialist clinics for late effects symptom management. One example is referral to a specialist gastroenterology clinic for effective diagnosis and treatment of diarrhoea lasting more than six months following pelvic radiotherapy.

Emotional needs

People who have cancer often express experiencing living with uncertainty. They may be having ongoing treatment, be under periodic surveillance, or have been told that the cancer is now cured or is incurable. This emotional roller coaster of a journey alongside the effects of the disease and treatment can impact profoundly on the individual's mental wellbeing. People can experience difficulty concentrating, insomnia, anxiety, depression, sexual problems, or lose confidence. About 45% of people with cancer express that the emotional effects of cancer are more difficult to cope with than the physical and practical aspects.

As guests in people's own homes, district nurses often see the signs when people are emotionally struggling. Asking open questions can help people to open up and express what is on their mind. There are a wide range of tactics available to support people with strengthening their coping mechanisms. These can vary from being there to listen, facilitating open family conversations, promoting the value of regular exercise, to signposting to local cancer support groups or self-management courses. If appropriate, individuals may benefit from a referral to the specialist palliative care team or being signposted to counselling.

Financial needs

The physical and emotional effects of cancer are the most common reasons people give up work or change jobs. Many people remain unaware of the benefits they may be entitled to for help with costs or the adaptations that may help in the workplace. Signposting individuals to benefits advice via Citizens Advice and the Macmillan Cancer Support helpline can facilitate suitable expert guidance (Figure 59.2).

Mental illness

Lesley Frater, QN

60

Box 60.1   Important factors that can trigger mental illness.

- Abuse
- Bereavement
- Conflict
- Chronic disease
- Genetic
- Major life events (good/bad)
- Social problems
- Substance abuse (drugs/alcohol)
- Medications (beta-blockers, codeine, morphine or steroids)

Box 60.2   Common screening tools.

- Patient Health Questionnaire (PHQ-9) https://patient.info/doctor/patient-health-questionnaire-phq-9
- Hospital Anxiety and Depression Scale (HAD)
- General Anxiety Disorder Scale https://patient.info/doctor/generalised-anxiety-disorder-assessment-gad-7

Box 60.3   Summary of the impacts of the Covid-19 pandemic on individual mental health.

Covid-19 Pandemic and Mental Health

- One of the biggest impacts to mental health ever experienced has been seen since the onset of the pandemic, which has affected people's mental health and wellbeing in different ways and at different points in time as the pandemic has progressed.
- The effects of social distancing, lockdown, the loss of loved ones to the virus and the over-consumption of stress-inducing media reports has taken a huge toll on the population's mental health and wellbeing; and will continue to have lasting effects long after the pandemic is over. (MIND, 2020)
- The publication 'Covid-19 and the nation's mental health' states that 10 million people (8.5 million adults and 1.5 million children and young people) in England will need support for their mental health as a direct result of the pandemic over the next three to five years (O'Shea 2021).
- People with experience of mental health problems are more likely to see their mental health worsen as a result of coronavirus restrictions (MIND, 2020)
- Drivers of worsening mental health during the pandemic include: social isolation, job and financial loss, housing insecurity, working in front-line services, loss of coping mechanisms, and reduced access to mental health services.

Mental illness is a term used to refer to a spectrum of mood disorders characterised by a sense of loss of control and subjective experiences of distress. In this chapter the term 'mental illness' is taken to include depression and anxiety conditions, the most common mental health conditions seen in primary care, often coexisting with chronic long-term physical illness. Mental ill health is the largest single cause of disability in the UK. It accounts for almost 23% of the overall burden of disease, compared to 16% each for cancer and cardiovascular disease.

Patients with chronic long-term health conditions have an increased risk of presenting with anxiety or depression. Other contributory factors include psychosocial problems, bereavement, chronic pain, emotional distress, onset of disability in previously healthy individuals, and physical changes making it more difficult for the body to adapt to stress (Box 60.1).

All nurses will at some time be in contact with people whose health is impaired, or quality of life is reduced due to mental health issues. Most community and primary care nurses are already playing an active role in supporting patients with mental health problems, but many have concerns about their ability to address these problems effectively.

Recognition of anxiety or anxiety with depression is crucial to patient care. If primary care staff do not have the knowledge to recognise the common symptoms, their ability to intervene will delay advice or referral to the appropriate health professional. Mental illness is not a normal part of the ageing process. It is a treatable medical illness, but if left unrecognised and untreated it can lead to disability, worsened chronic illnesses and ultimately suicide.

Clinical observations have revealed barriers to the effective management and treatment of mental health problems in people with or without chronic disease, including poor knowledge, fear, stigma and lack of relevant education in respect of commonly presenting mental illness.

Nurses working in the community and primary care need the requisite knowledge and to be educated to a level where they feel confident to recognise and manage commonly presenting mental health issues, whilst having the expertise to manage chronic illness. If nurses are to prevent suicide, they must be equipped to recognise and assess mental health problems when they first present (Box 60.2).

When a healthcare professional is presented with a patient who complains of symptoms of mental health illness, it is important that they consider all contributory factors such as psychological, social, cultural and physical characteristics and the quality of interpersonal relationships. They should consider the impact of these on the mental health symptoms and the implications for either referring onto appropriate services or preferred subsequent monitoring (Box 60.3).

Always ensure that as the healthcare professional you use jargon-free language when talking to patients and carers. It is important to ensure that shared decision-making takes place between patient and healthcare professionals in all aspects of care. It is very useful, where appropriate, to inform and offer patients, families and carers self-help management information, support groups and encourage them to participate in these programmes.

Common types of depression

- *Major depression*: A diagnosis of major depressive disorder is made if a person has five or more symptoms and impairment in usual functioning nearly every day during the same two-week period. Major depression often begins between ages 15 and 30 but also can appear in children. Episodes typically recur.
- *Reactive depression*: This is temporary and something everyone experiences. It alerts us that something may not quite be right in our lives and nudges us to reappraise aspects of our life that are not going well.
- *Anxiety with depression*: Depressed mood accompanied by any of the different types of anxiety.
- *Dysthymia*: People with this illness are mildly depressed for years. They function fairly well on a daily basis but over time their relationships suffer.
- *Bipolar disorder*: Mood changes back and forth between periods of depression and periods of mania (an extreme high). Less need for sleep, overconfidence, racing thoughts, reckless behaviour, increased energy, mood changes are usually gradual, but can be sudden.
- *Seasonal affective disorder (SAD)*: This is a depression that results from changes in the season. Most cases begin in the autumn or winter, or when there is a decrease in sunlight.

Common types of anxiety

- *Generalised anxiety disorder (GAD)*: Those affected worry about a number of things most days for six or more months. It usually affects young adults and women more than men. The anxiety is about a wide range of situations and issues.
- *Phobias*: These are extreme and irrational fears about a particular thing. The fears can be so great that the person goes to great lengths to avoid them, even if they are harmless.
- *Obsessive compulsive disorder (OCD)*: A person with OCD has unwanted, intrusive, persistent or repetitive thoughts, feelings, ideas or obsessions which cause anxiety. They then carry out actions to reduce the anxiety or get rid of those thoughts. For example, the person may be afraid of germs and try to relieve the anxiety by repeated handwashing.
- *Post-traumatic stress disorder (PTSD)*: This is a reaction to a highly stressful event outside the range of everyday experience such as war, violent attack (verbal, physical or sexual) or a natural disaster. The symptoms usually include irritability, anxiety, flashbacks, repeated nightmares and avoiding situations that might bring back memories of the event.
- *Panic disorder*: A person with a panic disorder has panic attacks. These are intense feelings of anxiety along with the kind of physical symptoms and overwhelming sensations of someone in great danger.

61 Assessing mental capacity

Beverly Graham, QN

Figure 61.1 A District Nurse speaks with an elderly man in his bed at home as part of a mental and physical health evaluation. Source: Courtesy of Matthew Peasey.

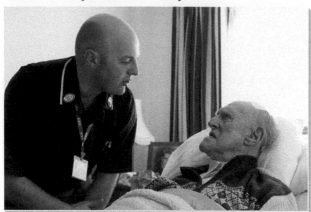

Figure 61.2 Patient-centred objectives of the Mental Capcity Act.

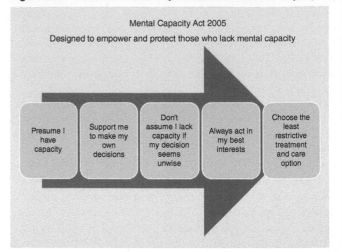

Mental Capacity Act 2005

Designed to empower and protect those who lack mental capacity

| Presume I have capacity | Support me to make my own decisions | Don't assume I lack capacity if my decision seems unwise | Always act in my best interests | Choose the least restrictive treatment and care option |

Box 61.1 Key principles of the Mental Capacity Act 2005.

- assume a person has the capacity to make a decision themselves, unless it's proved otherwise
- wherever possible, help people to make their own decisions
- do not treat a person as lacking the capacity to make a decision just because they make an unwise decision
- if you make a decision for someone who does not have capacity, it must be in their best interests

Treatment and care provided to someone who lacks capacity should be the least restrictive of their basic rights and freedoms.

Box 61.2 Helping people make their own decisions – factors to consider.

Factors to Consider:
- Helping people make their own decisions
- does the person have all the relevant information they need?
- have they been given information on any alternatives?
- could information be explained or presented in a way that's easier for them to understand (for example, by using simple language or visual aids)?
- have different methods of communication been explored, such as non-verbal communication?
- could anyone else help with communication, such as a family member, carer or advocate?
- are there particular times of day when the person's understanding is better?
- are there particular locations where the person may feel more at ease?
- could the decision be delayed until they might be better able to make the decision?

Further Information: https://www.nhs.uk/conditions/social-care-and-support-guide/making-decisions-for-someone-else/mental-capacity-act/

District Nursing at a Glance, First Edition. Edited by Matthew Bradby.
© 2022 John Wiley & Sons Ltd. Published 2022 by John Wiley & Sons Ltd.

Mental capacity is a person's ability to make decisions. This includes day-to-day decisions, for example what to eat, what to wear, and also more significant ones, for example the ability to make a decision that may have legal consequences, such as a will. A person should not be deemed to lack capacity simply because they make what others may deem an unwise decision.

What is meant by incapacity?

If a person has an impairment of, or disturbance in, the functioning of mind or brain, they are said to lack capacity. Impairment may be due to dementia, significant learning disabilities, brain damage, drowsiness, unconsciousness, or symptoms of drug and/or alcohol use. The loss of capacity could be partial or temporary. It is possible for a person to lack capacity to make one specific decision but not about another. People may be able to make everyday decisions but lack capacity to make complex decisions, such as those regarding financial affairs (Figure 61.1).

The Mental Capacity Act (2005)

The Mental Capacity Act (2005) provides the legal framework for making decisions on behalf of individuals who lack the mental capacity to make particular decisions themselves. The Act supports people who lack mental capacity and ensures that any decision or action is made in the person's best interests. It must be assumed that an adult over the age of 16 has the mental capacity to make decisions themselves unless shown otherwise at the time. This is referred to as 'presumption of capacity' (Figure 61.2).

The Act sets out five core principles for making decisions in relation to personal welfare, healthcare and financial matters affecting those who lack mental capacity. A person found guilty of ill treatment and/or neglect of a person who lacks capacity is liable to imprisonment for up to 5 years (Box 61.1).

Who should assess capacity?

Different people may be involved in assessing a person's capacity depending on the decision and when it needs to be made. In most instances this will be the main carer assisting with day-to-day decisions. Regarding healthcare decisions, it is up to the professional responsible for the person's treatment to ensure that capacity has been assessed.

What is the test of capacity?

There are two stages when assessing capacity:

Stage 1

Does the person have an impairment of, or a disturbance in the functioning of, their mind or brain? If the answer is 'No', they do not lack capacity under the Act. If the answer is 'Yes', proceed to stage 2.

Stage 2

Does the impairment or disturbance mean that the person is unable to make a specific decision when they need to?

In order to make a decision a person must be able to:

1 Understand the information relevant to the decision

Relevant information includes:

- The nature of the decision
- The reason why the decision is needed
- The effects of deciding one way or another, or making no decision at all.

It is important to take all possible steps to help people to understand and make a decision for themselves. A person with learning difficulties may need somebody to read information to them and offer an explanation. A person who does not speak English will need the help of an interpreter (Box 61.2).

2 Retain relevant information

The person must be able to retain the information given for long enough to use it to make the decision. If the person is able to retain the information relevant to a decision for a short period it should not automatically be assumed that they lack capacity to make the decision.

3 Weigh up the information

For someone to have capacity they must have the ability to weigh up information and use it to arrive at a decision. People may sometimes understand information but impairment may stop them from using it appropriately or may cause them to make impulsive decisions.

4 Communicate the decision

People may be unable to speak but may communicate in other ways (e.g. blinking or writing). Sometimes there is no way for a person to communicate, for example during unconsciousness or coma. If a person is unable to communicate their decision despite all assistance they should be treated as unable to make a decision. Treatment or actions must be carried out as best interests.

Making decisions in a person's best Interests

- The person must be involved in making the decision and given any help they need to take part.
- All the relevant circumstances must be considered; for example, what might they have wanted if they had capacity?
- It is essential to respect religious beliefs and culture.
- Do not make assumptions about what the person wants just because of their age, appearance, condition or behaviour.
- Consider whether they are likely to gain capacity.
- Consult with others who know the person well (e.g. family, friends, carers, and other professionals).
- Try to limit restrictions on the person's decision.

Lasting power of attorney and enduring power of attorney

Lasting power of attorney (LPA) is a legal document allowing a chosen person to make decisions for another (which must be in the person's best interests). It was introduced with the Mental Capacity Act and replaced enduring power of attorney (EPA), which only covered property and financial affairs.

There are two types of LPA:

- Health and welfare
- Property and financial affairs.

A person can choose to make one type or both.

Professional record-keeping

Healthcare professionals should record capacity assessments, findings, decisions and treatment in the relevant professional records as part of individual care planning processes. Nurses may be guided by the Nursing and Midwifery Council (NMC) Code.

Dementia

Morejoy Saineti, QN

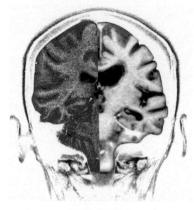

Figure 62.1 Healthy brain (left); advanced Alzheimer's (right). Source: Science History Images/Alamy Stock Photo.

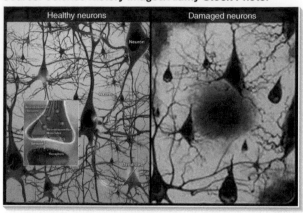

Figure 62.2 Comparison of healthy and damaged neurons. Source: Science History Images/Alamy Stock Photo.

Figure 62.4 Haemorrhagic and ischaemic stroke. Source: Types of Stroke, Heart and Stroke Foundation of Canada. © 2020 Heart and Stroke Foundation of Canada.

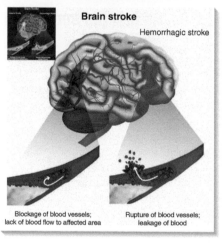

Figure 62.3 Arterial supply to the brain, showing capillaries. Source: Gandee Vasan/Getty Images.

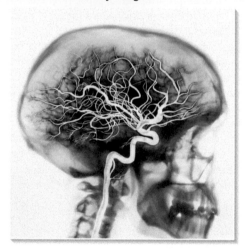

Figure 62.5 Dementia with Lewy bodies.

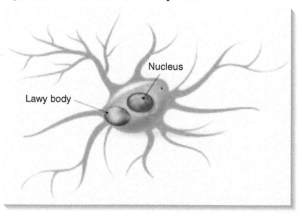

According to the World Health Organization, dementia is a syndrome caused by brain disease, usually of a chronic or progressive nature, in which there is disturbance of multiple higher cortical functions, including memory, thinking, orientation, comprehension, calculation, learning capacity, language and judgement. There are several hundred types of dementia classified according to the conditions causing the dementia and the area of the brain affected (Figures 62.1 and 62.2).

Alzheimer's disease

Alzheimer's is the most common type of dementia, affecting half of people with dementia. There are more than 520,000 people in the UK with Alzheimer's disease. Proteins build up in the brain to form structures called 'plaques' and 'tangles'. This results in loss of connections between nerve cells, progressing to the death of nerve cells and loss of brain tissue. Alzheimer's is associated with shortage of some important chemicals which help to transmit signals around the brain. Current treatments for Alzheimer's disease help boost the levels of chemical messengers in the brain, reducing the symptoms.

Two types of medication are used to treat Alzheimer's disease: acetylcholinesterase inhibitors (cholinesterase inhibitors) and NMDA receptor antagonists. The generic names for the cholinesterase inhibitors are donepezil (Aricept), rivastigmine (Exelon), and galantamine (Reminyl XL, Acumor XL, Galsya XL and Gatalin XL). The NMDA receptor antagonist is memantine (Ebixa, Maruxa and Nemdatine).

Vascular dementia

In the case of vascular dementia, blood supply to the brain is damaged in some way (Figure 62.3). In multi-infarct dementia tiny strokes cut off the blood supply to small areas of the brain, resulting in cell death. Recent research has shown that smoking is a significant risk factor for vascular dementia and Alzheimer's, with smokers twice as likely to develop the disease as non-smokers. Some of the other underlying risk factors are high cholesterol levels, obesity, high blood pressure and diabetes. To be healthy and function properly, brain cells need a constant supply of blood to bring oxygen and nutrients. If the vascular system within the brain becomes damaged, with the blood vessels leaking or becoming blocked, then blood cannot reach the brain cells and they will eventually die (Figure 62.4). Progression of vascular disease may happen in a step-like way.

If the underlying cardiovascular diseases that have caused vascular dementia can be controlled, it may be possible to slow down the progression of the dementia. For example, after someone has had a stroke or transient ichaemic attack, treatment of high blood pressure can reduce the risk of further stroke and dementia. In most cases, a person with vascular dementia will already be on medications to treat the underlying diseases. These include tablets to reduce blood pressure, prevent blood clots and lower cholesterol.

If the person has a diagnosed heart condition or diabetes they will also be taking medicines for these. It is important that the person continues to take any medications and attends regular check-ups as recommended by a doctor. Adopting a healthy lifestyle with regular physical exercise, a healthy weight, low alcohol intake, and quitting smoking helps to reduce the risk. A diet with plenty of fruit, vegetables and oily fish but not too much fat or salt is helpful.

Lewy body dementia

Lewy body dementia shares symptoms with both Alzheimer's disease and Parkinson's disease. It accounts for around 10% of all cases of dementia. Dementia with Lewy bodies (DLB) tends to be mistakenly diagnosed as other conditions and thus is underdiagnosed. Lewy bodies are tiny deposits of protein in nerve cells (Figure 62.5). The disease is marked with hallucination, distress or disturbed behaviour, perception problems, and a patient prone to falls and sleep problems.

Rarer causes of dementia

Frontotemporal lobe dementia

This term covers a range of specific conditions. It is sometimes called Pick's disease or frontal lobe dementia. Frontotemporal dementia is caused when nerve cells in the frontal and/or temporal lobes of the brain die and the pathways that connect them change. There is also some loss of important chemical messengers. The brain tissue in the frontal and temporal lobes shrinks over time. Symptoms include changes in personality and behaviour, and difficulties with language, as well as marked disinhibition.

Creutzfeldt–Jakob disease

Creutzfeldt–Jakob disease (CJD) is caused by an abnormally shaped protein called a prion infecting the brain. Sporadic CJD, which normally affects people over 40, is the most common form of the disease. CJD affects about one out of every 1 million people each year. It is not known what triggers sporadic CJD.

HIV-associated neurocognitive disorder

HIV (human immunodeficiency virus) makes it harder for the body to fight infections and disease. It can cause a number of different problems in the brain, affecting up to half of people with HIV. This is known as HIV-associated neurocognitive disorder (HAND). Before the use of antiretroviral drugs, around 20–30% of people with advanced HIV infection previously developed dementia, but this has now decreased to around 2%. Neurocognitive disorders may be caused by the HIV virus directly damaging the brain, with the weakened immune system also enabling other infectious agents to attack brain cells. Symptoms include problems with short-term memory, learning, speed of thinking, difficulties with concentration and decision-making, unsteadiness and mood changes and problems with the sense of smell.

Learning disability

Raj Jhamat, QN and Shirley Chappel, QN

Figure 63.1   Example of a hospital passport.

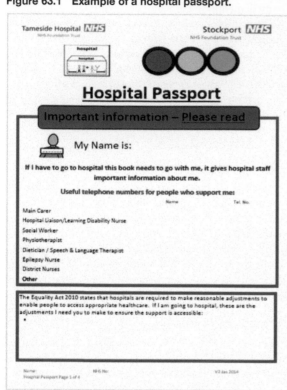

District Nursing at a Glance, First Edition. Edited by Matthew Bradby.
© 2022 John Wiley & Sons Ltd. Published 2022 by John Wiley & Sons Ltd.

A learning disability has been described as 'a significant reduced ability to understand new or complex information, to learn new skills (*impaired intelligence*), with a reduced ability to cope independently (*impaired social functioning*) which started before adulthood, with a lasting effect on development' (Valuing People White Paper, Department of Health, 2001). A learning disability is an intellectual functioning level well below average, usually with an IQ below 70, as well as significant limitations in two or more adaptive skill areas.

'Adaptive skills' refer to skills needed by people for daily life such as:

- Understanding language, other people, and the world around them
- Expressing themselves
- Understanding, managing and expressing their feelings
- Building and maintaining relationships
- Keeping themselves safe
- Looking after their personal hygiene, health, and nutrition
- Learning and remembering.

The term learning disability is often confused with 'learning difficulty', possibly because they both have an effect on intellect. A learning difficulty concerns a narrow area of learning and so it tends to affect specific areas of your life, such as reading and writing (e.g. dyslexia). People with dyslexia do not tend to have a general difficulty with learning in other areas of life, so do not have a learning disability.

Community learning disability teams

Community learning disability teams (CLDT) are multidisciplinary teams that provide an in-depth specialist assessment of people with learning disabilities who have complex physical and health needs. This leads to the delivery and coordination of person-centred care packages, a personalised agenda, and improvement to overall health and wellbeing.

The teams will differ depending on the population needs in each area, but usually they will include learning disability nurses, physiotherapists, speech and language therapists, occupational therapists, psychologists and social workers. One of the key roles of any CLDT is to support and prepare individuals with learning disabilities to access secondary care settings (alongside their carers, family or other professionals) through admission and discharge meetings. In some CLDTs this is supported and guided by a hospital liaison nurse.

Hospital liaison nurse

A hospital liaison nurse (HLN) is available to support people with learning disabilities who are going into hospital. Their role is to work with people to help them to understand why they are going to hospital and what will happen while they are there. They can, in some situations, support the person with 'desensitisation' to help them to be more concordant with treatment and to avoid unnecessary distress.

Not everyone who has a learning disability will be able to understand their treatment and give informed consent for procedures. The HLN is available to support other professionals in assessing patients' understanding and ability to consent under the Mental Capacity Act 2005. For those people who are unable to consent, they will support staff with making best-interest decisions.

The HLN will work in close partnership with the person who has learning disabilities, family and carers, and hospital staff to plan and make sure that all the person's needs are met from admission to discharge. In many situations, this involves advising hospital staff around 'reasonable adjustments' that they can make to their usual service to make this more person-centred and accessible for the individual. They will also provide regular training sessions for hospital staff on how to support people with learning disabilities. A HLN may be located either within the CLDTs or within the hospital itself. It is useful to know where your local HLN is based and how to contact them.

National and local guidance recommends that all people with learning disabilities have a hospital passport that accompanies them whenever they are being admitted to hospital (Figure 63.1). A hospital passport is usually completed in an easier read format and provides a description of the whole person, not only information about illness and health. It should also include information regarding a person's likes or dislikes, from physical contact to their favourite type of drink, as well as their interests and preferred communication style – for example, if they use British Sign Language. This will help all the hospital staff know how to make people feel more comfortable and will provide a guide in ensuring they receive the right support during their stay. The hospital passport should be completed with full involvement of the person who has learning disabilities and their families/carers. They are available from local CLDTs or hospitals.

People with learning disabilities who have been an inpatient in a hospital setting should also have a discharge plan in place to allow for a smooth transition back home and to identify any ongoing support needs. The information contained in this plan should include:

- What the person was treated for and if they have a new or additional diagnosis with different support needs.
- Does the person need any extra equipment, and if so, who will buy it?
- Do they staff team need training in any procedures, and if so, who will provide it?
- Is there a change to the person's medication?
- Are there any follow-up appointments?
- Are there any pressure areas?
- Is the information included in the health action plan?

The discharge planning process should be completed with full involvement of the person who has learning disabilities and their families or carers, and the acute staff. The discharge paperwork should be available from local HLNs or hospital trusts.

For further information about the work of Community Learning Disability Nurses, see chapter 67.

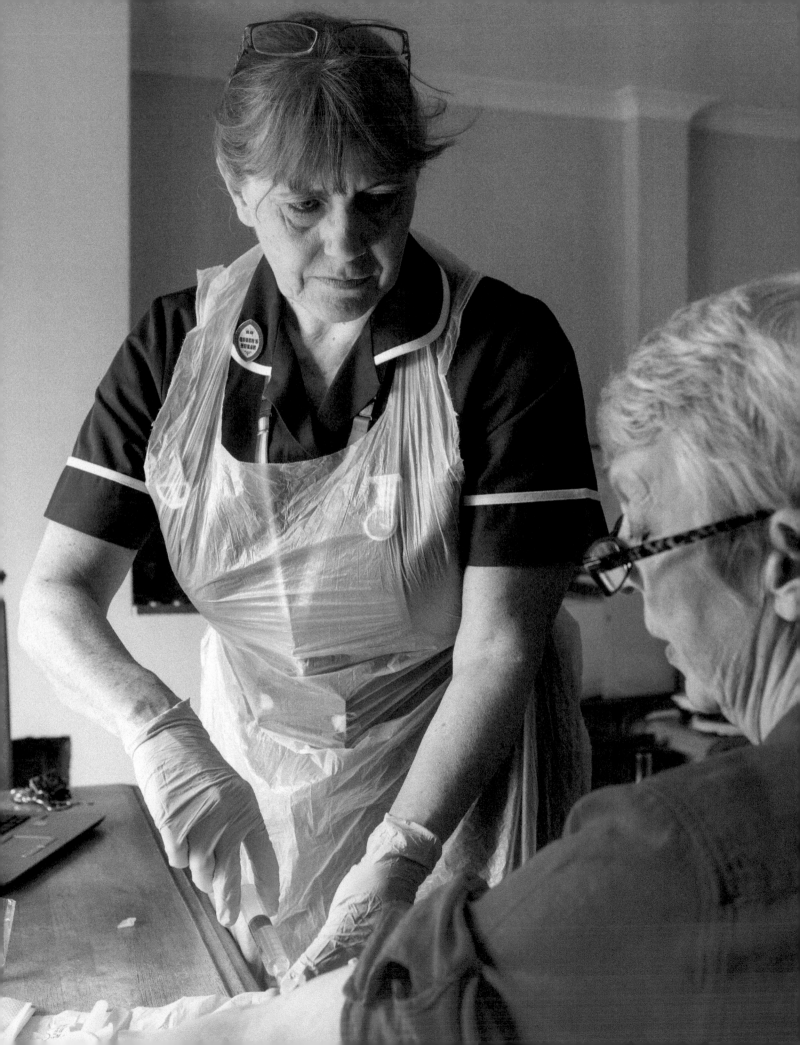

Specialisms in the community

Part 6

Chapters

64 Specialist nurses and the role of district nurses in coordinating care

Sadie Campbell, QN

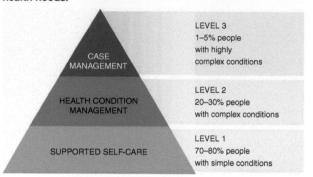

Figure 64.1   Kaiser Permanente triangle of population-based health needs.

- **CASE MANAGEMENT** — LEVEL 3 / 1–5% people with highly complex conditions
- **HEALTH CONDITION MANAGEMENT** — LEVEL 2 / 20–30% people with complex conditions
- **SUPPORTED SELF-CARE** — LEVEL 1 / 70–80% people with simple conditions

Box 64.1   Case management: main principles of case management.

- Single point of contact
- Assessment of need
- Tailored individualised care pathways
- Orchestration of services
- Coordinating care
- Independent prescribing
- Carer support
- Facilitating early discharge
- Avoiding unnecessary admissions
- Managing acute exacerbations

Box 64.2   Key skills.

- Accurate nursing assessment
- Reassessment of nursing needs
- Identifying and managing risk
- Orchestration of services
- Coordinating of care
- Integrated working
- Effective communication skills
- Acting as a patient advocate

Box 64.3   Care management: main principles of care management.

- Case finding
- Screening
- Assessment of need
- Care planning
- Monitoring of care plan
- Review of care needs
- Integrated working

District Nursing at a Glance, First Edition. Edited by Matthew Bradby.
© 2022 John Wiley & Sons Ltd. Published 2022 by John Wiley & Sons Ltd.

istrict nurses work with family members, GPs, allied health professionals, carers and community groups to meet an individual's needs and to coordinate their care. By so doing, they improve individuals' quality of life and help them remain independent for as long as possible, managing long-term conditions and sometimes their end-of-life care. Increasingly, the trend is towards personalised care – a negotiated process between patient and clinician that seeks to identify and meet the needs and desires of the patient in their care plan.

Core role of the district nurse

District nurses play a pivotal role in community healthcare today, adapting to the changing needs of patients and the demands of healthcare. The core of district nursing is based on the nursing process; district nurses need to be skilled at assessing, planning, implementing and evaluating patient care needs. They play a crucial role in the primary healthcare team and also participate as members of the wider healthcare community. They are ideally placed to coordinate a significant part of the patient journey, implementing strategies that keep patients in their own home for as long as possible. With fewer hospital beds available, quicker discharges and patients choosing to stay at home for longer and in many cases to die at home, the role of the district nurse will only become more essential, as has been amply demonstrated during the Covid-19 pandemic. Being able to care for patients wishing to live and die in their own homes can be a moving and rewarding experience.

Nursing is multifaceted and ever-changing and it is therefore essential to ensure that skills and knowledge are kept up to date. District nurses remain patient-focused whether they are managing difficult cases or organising general caseload management, making clinical decisions or teaching students. Community nursing also requires a whole-family approach and involving the patient and their family is essential. Informal carers play an indispensable role and community nurses have a vital role as advocates for carers. As patients' nursing needs become ever more complex, nurses have to develop and extend their skills, but still need to remain focused on the baseline of good nursing care. Nursing means caring for patients, starting with the basics, getting a proper nursing assessment completed, and ensuring that personalised care plans are in place, with the patient's informed consent.

It is recognised that district nursing can be seen as a complex field of practice. There are a huge variety of roles within community nursing from case management, care management, risk assessment, specialist roles to teaching and mentorship. Nurses work with patients at all levels (Figure 64.1). Being a mentor is also a valuable and rewarding role for nurses and helps students progress their career pathway. Good leadership is also essential for the district nursing profession to have a clear vision for the future. Nursing is adaptable to change and continuous professional development enables nurses to enhance their knowledge and skills to give the most up-to-date care, yielding best outcomes for patients.

Regular supervision and reflective practice is beneficial for nurses to help them develop themselves professionally.

Working with specialist nurses and services

District nurses coordinate services, referrals and joint visits with social workers, occupational therapists, hospice nurses, GPs, Marie Curie nurses and other specialists as normal practice. Working in partnership with specialist nurses is more likely to lead to better patient outcomes. Specialist nurses and district nurses work in partnership with patients, families and carers to:

- provide skilled nursing care at home;
- promote and maintain patient independence; and
- provide patient education and advice and support self-management.

The district nurse often has specialist interests (Box 64.1). They oversee the care of patients with long-term conditions and work with disease-specific nurse specialists, who are an enormous support for district nurses with their knowledge and contacts. Specialist nurses have direct access to disease-specific consultants in acute settings and are able to get information quickly for district nurses to help with symptom management (Box 64.2). Integrated care with specialists has also been a vital part of the response to Covid-19.

Examples of specialist nurses in community care

- Continence nurses
- Tissue viability nurses
- Heart function nurse specialists
- Respiratory nurse specialists
- Diabetic nurse specialists
- Hospice nurses
- Acute care at home nursing teams
- Case managers
- Nurse practitioners
- Care managers (Box 64.3).

Summary

District nurses and their teams can care for many patients experiencing exacerbations of their long-term condition, avoiding unnecessary hospital admissions. District nursing teams also provide a seamless transition of care service from hospital to community care, and are central to integrated services that 'wrap around' the patient, giving the most appropriate care when it is most needed. District nursing encompasses care within the home, delivering patient choice and supporting the integration of general practice, hospital care and the wider health and social care network. As NHS policy seeks to keep patients at home for as long as possible, reduce hospital admissions and facilitate early discharge, district nurses and their teams are ideally placed to enable this. In 2020, the support and rehabilitation in the community of people recovering from Covid-19 has become an additional major responsibility.

65 Voluntary organisations and district nurses

Carol Singleton, QN

Table 65.1 What sort of voluntary organisations could be useful to district nurses?

Name	Subject area	Website
Campaigning groups		
Diabetes UK	Fighting to ensure that everyone affected by diabetes gets access to the best standards of care/treatment	www.diabetes.org.uk/
Multiple Sclerosis Society	Fighting to improve treatment and care to help people with MS take control of their lives	www.mssociety.org.uk/
Age UK	Working towards a world where older people have opportunities to participate in society and enjoy life, as much as possible, for as long as possible	www.ageuk.org.uk/
Carers Trust	Provide access to desperately needed breaks, information and advice and education, training and employment opportunities	www.carers.org
Social or healthcare providers		
British Red Cross	Support at home, short-term loan mobility aids, reablement admission avoidance, A&E support, assisted discharge	www.redcross.org.uk/en
Information-giving organisations		
Macmillan	Resources for Cancer sufferers, carers, family and professionals	www.macmillan.org.uk/
Diabetes UK	Guides to diabetes, resources for people with diabetes, families and professionals	www.diabetes.org.uk/
Parkinson's UK	Information leaflets. Confidential support helpline	www.parkinsons.org.uk/
Alzheimer's Society	Confidential support helpline	www.alzheimers.org.uk/
Citizens Advice Bureaux	Free, independent, confidential and impartial advice online, by phone or in person at a local Citizens Advice centre. Help people resolve their problems with benefits, work, debt and money, consumer, discrimination	www.citizensadvice.org.uk/about-us/how-we-provide-advice/advice/Get-advice/
MIND	Support and information on services, money and benefits, relating to mental health.	www.mind.org.uk
Stroke Association	Provides high-quality, up-to-date stroke information for stroke patients, their families and carers	www.stroke.org.uk/
Support groups		
Macmillan	Cancer sufferers, carers, family. info centres, buddy service	www.macmillan.org.uk/
British Red Cross	First aid courses, transport, hand, arm and shoulder massage, teaching resources	www.redcross.org.uk/en
Parkinson's UK	13 teams across UK providing support and information, give training on parkinsons	www.parkinsons.org.uk/
Multiple Sclerosis Society	Provides emotional support, benefits guidance and help to get the right care	www.mssociety.org.uk/
Alzheimer's Society	Resources and training, for people with Alzheimer's, carers and professionals	www.alzheimers.org.uk/
Age UK	Handyperson services, home shopping delivery, exercise classes, lunch clubs	www.ageuk.org.uk/
Royal Voluntary Service	Meals on wheels, community transport, befriending	www.royalvoluntaryservice.org.uk/
Epilepsy Action	Resources, advice and information on living with epilepsy	www.epilepsy.org.uk
MENCAP	Works with people with a learning disability to change laws, challenge prejudice and support them to live their lives as they choose	www.mencap.org.uk
Asthma UK	Fund research, campaign to improve quality of care and provide advice and support	www.asthma.org.uk
Carers UK	Resources, information, support, search for local information, campaign for carers.	www.carersuk.org/
Remap	Design and make bespoke equipment to help people carry out essential daily tasks or take part in leisure or sporting activities.	www.remap.org.uk/about-us/

District Nursing at a Glance, First Edition. Edited by Matthew Bradby.
© 2022 John Wiley & Sons Ltd. Published 2022 by John Wiley & Sons Ltd.

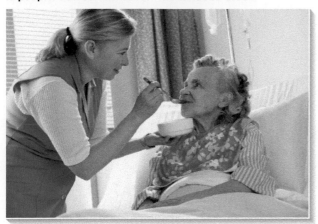

Figure 65.1   Voluntary services provide vital companionship to people. Source: Alexander Raths/Adobe Stock.

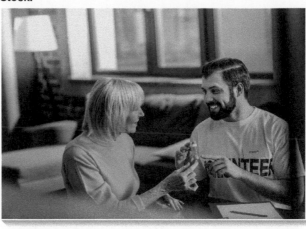

Figure 65.2   Voluntary services support people at home, including care homes. Source: Viacheslav Lakobchuk/Adobe Stock.

The largest number of patients making up the district nurse's caseload will be adults of all ages with long-term conditions, including multiple sclerosis, asthma, cystic fibrosis, diabetes, paralysis, to older people with conditions that develop as a result of natural ageing. The challenge for healthcare professionals is to meet an individual's specific needs, not necessarily exclusively themselves but by working in conjunction with other appropriate professionals and organisations, and also to ensure that their carers receive all the support and advice they may need.

What is a voluntary organisation?

A voluntary organisation is an organisation that is composed of or functions with the aid of volunteers and which provides aid or services to individuals and/or groups. It is a term used to describe those organisations that focus on wider public benefit, rather than statutory service delivery or profit. They are also known as 'third sector' or not-for-profit organisations. There are different types of voluntary groups: campaigning groups, social or healthcare providers, information-giving organisations and support groups.

There can be as many as 500 distinct voluntary organisations operating in any one area and these will probably not all be mapped according to the services they provide. This can make the district nurse's job much more challenging when seeking support or services for a patient. As most organisations have a website, an online search can help to narrow the possible opportunities available, which can then be explored in more detail. Additionally, some local authorities provide print or online information on the services provided in their area.

A patient may need more help with everyday living, or support in the home (Figure 65.1). Healthcare staff may need information for themselves, the patient or carer, on a specific condition or disease, treatment or help, access to respite care, advice about their finances, or help with accessing specialist equipment. The voluntary organisations most commonly used by district nurses are Marie Curie, Macmillan, Age UK, the Alzheimer's Society, British Red Cross and local hospices.

Before the introduction of the internet, the only medium available to district nurses to share information with their patients and their carers was leaflets or telephone contacts. Now most families can access the internet themselves or through friends and family members and this should be encouraged. However it is useful if nurses can provide a brief list of possible websites to help initiate the process.

Well-informed patients and their carers will feel more engaged with their care, able to ask questions of their healthcare professionals and able to gain support from other individuals living with similar health conditions to enable them to participate in planning their ongoing and future care (Figure 65.2).

Voluntary organisations can make all the difference to how a patient and their carers continue to manage at home and should always form part of the district nurse's toolbox when considering problems associated with finances, information, support or equipment. They should be viewed as additional members of the team and working in partnership with them can be of enormous benefit to nurses, patients and carers (Table 65.1).

Occupational health: specialist community public health nurses

Catherine Best, QN

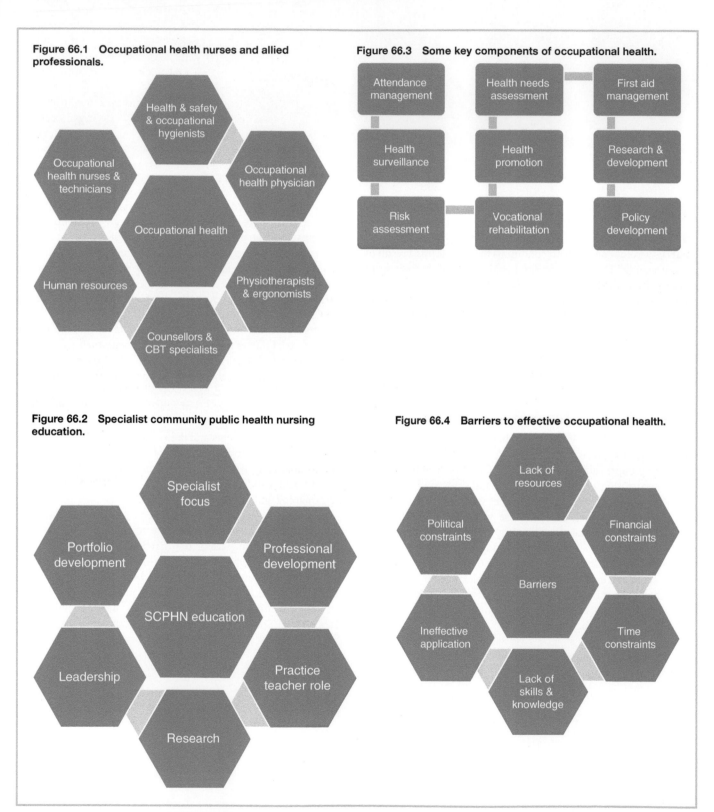

Figure 66.1 Occupational health nurses and allied professionals.

- Health & safety & occupational hygienists
- Occupational health nurses & technicians
- Occupational health physician
- Occupational health
- Human resources
- Physiotherapists & ergonomists
- Counsellors & CBT specialists

Figure 66.3 Some key components of occupational health.

- Attendance management
- Health needs assessment
- First aid management
- Health surveillance
- Health promotion
- Research & development
- Risk assessment
- Vocational rehabilitation
- Policy development

Figure 66.2 Specialist community public health nursing education.

- Specialist focus
- Portfolio development
- Professional development
- SCPHN education
- Leadership
- Practice teacher role
- Research

Figure 66.4 Barriers to effective occupational health.

- Lack of resources
- Political constraints
- Financial constraints
- Barriers
- Ineffective application
- Time constraints
- Lack of skills & knowledge

District Nursing at a Glance, First Edition. Edited by Matthew Bradby.
© 2022 John Wiley & Sons Ltd. Published 2022 by John Wiley & Sons Ltd.

Specialist role

There is currently a very diverse range of roles within occupational health, including occupational health advisors, nurses and technicians. It is the role of the specialist community public health nurses (SCPHN), however, to develop strategies based on the health needs of the working population and to directly influence policies that affect health. Specifically, SCPHNs working in occupational health focus on the provision of advice to those in the workplace setting.

SCPHNs work across professional disciplines (Figure 66.1) to ensure employees remain suitable for the role to which they are deployed, providing support strategies which, if utilised effectively, can actively promote and protect the health and wellbeing of the working age population. Utilising a multitude of paradigms including evidence-based practice, current legislation and sector-specific standards, the specialism of occupational health is now primarily driven by confident and accountable SCPHNs who are not afraid to challenge the status quo.

It could be argued that public health nursing includes the role of the district nurse, working for the betterment of both individuals and populations, demonstrating that as a community of healthcare professionals, we are working towards the same overall aims. Critically analysing the role of district nurses and SCPHNs working in occupational health, it is evident that there is some overlap between their roles, not least that they work to improve outcomes for those individuals who are undergoing rehabilitation, including neurology, drug and alcohol misuse, musculoskeletal disorders and mental health.

The working population may be a smaller part of the district nurse's current caseload depending upon demographics; however, with lifestyle changes meaning that people are living increasingly longer with chronic health conditions, it is likely that the burden of chronic disease will become increasingly prevalent in the working age population.

Synergistic working

Although there is no legal requirement to complete an academic course in this specialist field, completion of the SCPHN course in occupational health is seen as a 'gateway' to developing skills which have the ability to influence practice at a senior level. Education does not cease with the SCPHN course, as there exist a multitude of further opportunities to develop other specialist skills (Figure 66.2).

The role of the SCPHN is a complex and multifaceted one, the management of which requires the development of strong and effective working relationships across a wide range of roles based on a level of openness, professional integrity and governance, autonomous practice and self-belief (Figure 66.3). It is evident that many of these roles can be identified as those similar to that of a district nurse. By taking a critical approach to their role, it is possible for a district nurse to visualise their defined 'population' in the broadest sense. For example, involving local employers and other agencies, a nurse may accomplish significantly more than can be achieved by working alone.

Consider, for example, the patient who is currently absent from work following major surgery, where the district nurse is involved with aftercare (e.g. dressing changes and assessing milestones of recovery). The aim of the district nurse is likely to be focused on the patient making a full recovery, whereas the main aim of the patient, however, may simply be to become fit enough to return to work. This understanding by the district nurse is more likely to encourage communication with a member of the occupational health team who can develop a rehabilitation programme using a collaborative approach with workplace management. This approach has the potential to enable an employee to return to work promptly, albeit perhaps to a less demanding role or with recuperative hours in the short term. The resulting reduction of the potential financial stressor is likely to further enable recovery, creating a win–win situation for employer and employee as well as role satisfaction for the clinicians. The potential barrier to such synergistic working is the important one of confidentiality in relation to sharing of information; however, this is easily overcome by the effective use of informed consent as early as possible in the process and full involvement of the patient throughout.

Future expectations

The progressive role of the SCPHN and the district nurse will require the ability to work in a rapidly changing environment, demonstrating effective leadership, implementing change and integrating national policy at a local level. Community nurses of all disciplines will be central to the implementation of future government and professional policy, being required to work in an increasingly collaborative manner to form partnerships that will help improve outcomes for local populations, whether of working age or beyond. It is evident that the shape of our society is changing. This requires all community nurses to be flexible and adaptable to working within partnerships to enable the best outcomes for individuals. How these challenges are faced will determine the fate of our professions as a whole, as well as that of the populations within our communities.

Crucially, district nurses and SCPHNs working in occupational health are likely to become increasingly significant players in healthcare provision as services continue to move into those communities. This is a challenging time for all healthcare professionals with barriers (resourcing, financial and political) suggesting that there is a long way to go (Figure 66.4). These barriers can be overcome by seizing every opportunity to work collaboratively and work towards establishing synergies as a fundamental aspect of community healthcare reform.

67 Community learning disability nursing

Denise Souter, QN

Figure 67.1 Community learning disability nurses may provide health education to those they work with. Source: Learning disability and dementia.

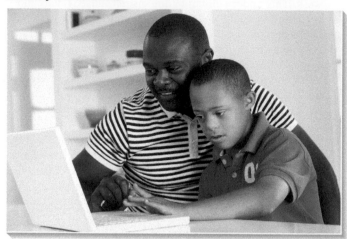

Figure 67.3 A young man with learning disabilities being supported to undertake outdoor activities.

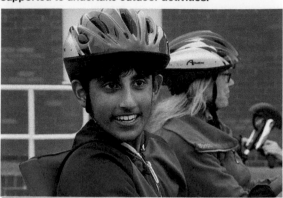

Figure 67.2 National Health Service Covid-19 Grab and Go Guide for people with learning disabilities and autism. NHS England and NHS Improvement coronavirus, https://www.england.nhs.uk/coronavirus/wp-content/uploads/sites/52/2020/03/C0381-nhs-covid-19-grab-and-go-lda-form.pdf. Licensed under Open Government Licence v3.0.

COVID-19 Grab and Go guide
Form

NHS

I have a learning disability or I am autistic

⚠️

- **This guide is really important during the COVID-19 pandemic**
- The Human Rights Act means that staff in the NHS must respect and protect my human rights when making decisions about my care even in the time of the COVID-19 pandemic.
- Decisions about treatment should be made on an individual basis and in consultation with families, taking into account my usual health. Decisions about my treatment and resuscitation should not be made based on my learning disability or autism or the Clinical Frailty Scale.
- All decisions must be made in accordance with the principles of the Mental Capacity Act.

My name is:

I like to be called: Date of birth:

My NHS Number is:

My next of kin/representative:

Their phone number:

I am able to indicate YES and NO to your questions by:

I have previously had the following breathing problems (asthma/history of infections, etc):

Any other things that may comprise my airway, e.g. past surgery:

What you need to know about my other past and current health (e.g. diabetes / epilepsy):

I usually take the following medication (include dose of tablets or liquid or any other way I take medicine):

This is the help I need to understand what is happening and the support I may need with any treatment:

Swallowing and oral care, including how I drink (e.g. small amounts or thickened or cooled, or any other way I need to take it):   ☐ No issues   ☐ Detail below

This is how people usually know if I am in pain:

If I'm worried or upset I may:

I communicate by:

My hearing and my eyesight (e.g. hearing aids, glasses or anything else I need to help me hear or see):

This should be read in conjunction with my hospital passport

On average, the life expectancy of women with a learning disability is 18 years shorter than in the general population and for men with a learning disability it is 14 years shorter than in the general population (NHS Digital, 2017).

Reports from Disability Rights Commission and the charity Mencap have emphasised the need to tackle the health inequalities of people with a learning disability. Community learning disability nurses have been identified as being best placed to help promote access to mainstream health services providing specialist support, working to reduce barriers and educating allied health professionals. They are one of the specialists whose role is often coordinated in partnership with the district nurse and other members of the multidisciplinary team.

The focus of the community learning disability nurse is to provide care and support to children and adults with a learning disability, to enable a healthy and good quality of life with as much independence as possible (Figure 67.1). Part of their role is also to ensure that the person with a learning disability has opportunities to reach their full potential without prejudice. The nursing care is person-centred, with all areas of health being assessed and evaluated with a holistic approach, whilst supporting positive self-image and social inclusion. The community learning disability nurse acts as an advocate and a voice for the person with a learning disability whilst recognising contributions of family and carers. They support the person with learning difficulties in a full range of settings including their own home, in school, in residential community centres, in hospital, in mental health settings, and even in prison (Figure 67.2).

Some examples of the work of a community learning disability nurse include:

- Assessing and planning care and writing a care plan
- Teaching people with a learning disability basic life skills and how to keep safe within the community ('stranger danger' awareness)
- Liaising with care professionals, relatives and social care teams
- Monitoring health and formulating health action plans
- Risk management
- Enabling self-advocacy and promoting self-worth
- Promoting good health (coordinating and running health groups, ensuring uptake of general health checks)
- Monitoring mental health (taking on the role as care coordinator)
- Communication facilitator (this would include ensuring that the person with a learning disability has access to any easy read information to meet their needs with understanding information)

- Monitoring medications/side effects
- Safeguarding awareness/attending meeting and being alert to any concerns
- Workshop training for people with a learning disability, their family and any professionals
- Referral to other professionals if required
- Providing support to relatives and carers.

Working as a community learning disability nurse gives opportunities to make a huge difference to a person with learning difficulty (Figure 67.3).

Case study

A community learning disability nurse was tasked to support and coordinate the care of a man with Down's syndrome who was dying of liver cancer, and to give support his family. The patient was very scared of healthcare settings due to adverse experience of previous hospital care, and so doctors, nurses and services were struggling to care for him effectively, causing concern to both professionals and family. Part of the care plan was therefore to build up a therapeutic relationship with the patient (and his mother), facilitating a smooth pathway for his palliative care, as required. The nurse in this case needed to work closely in partnership with all professionals involved, with the patient and his mother.

To overcome the patient's fear of professionals, the nurse asked the man about his likes and dislikes and found that he had a love of music. He also liked pottery and horse riding as well as the television programme *Doctor Who*. It was agreed with the hospice, hospital and palliative care nurses that the man would attend the pottery art group at the hospice and he would also have his checkups and medical appointments there. This would avoid attending hospital, as nearly all his monitoring and treatment could be done at the hospice. In this case, the man got to know and trust the staff at the hospice and he called his medical appointments 'going to pottery'. The nurse played music when travelling to appointments, which reduced the patient's stress and made the treatment pathway as tolerable, even pleasant, as possible. Eventually the man passed away in the hospice with his pottery and artwork in his room. The hospice nurses and his family were with him and he had a peaceful death.

This example highlights good practice and how nursing in the community can be diverse and rewarding. It also highlights the importance of person-centred care and establishing what is important to every individual in their healthcare, at whatever stage of life.

Tuberculosis nursing

Nicky Brown, QN and Simone Thorn Heathcock, QN

Figure 68.1   A chest x-ray of a TB patient. Source: tbalert, www.tbalert.org

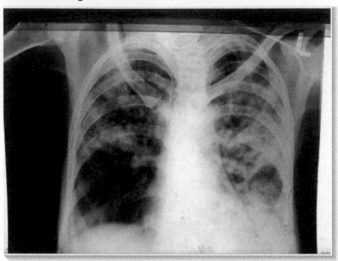

Figure 68.2   Key actions to eliminate TB.

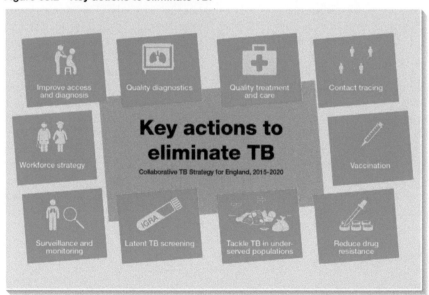

District Nursing at a Glance, First Edition. Edited by Matthew Bradby.
© 2022 John Wiley & Sons Ltd. Published 2022 by John Wiley & Sons Ltd.

Tuberculosis (TB) is a communicable disease most commonly caused by infection with the bacillus *Mycobacterium tuberculosis*. Other mycobacteria can also cause TB, such as *M. bovis*, *M. africanum* and *M. canettii*. TB can be present in any part of the body but most commonly affects the lungs, and is only infectious if it is pulmonary. TB is notifiable in the UK under the Health Protection (Part 2A Orders) Regulations 2010.

Epidemiology

There are over nine million new infections with TB globally every year, and around 1.7 million deaths. The UK has an infection rate of 12.3/100,000 people with TB, and urban areas such as London have even higher numbers. Much of the TB in the UK is seen in people born outside of the UK (73%).

Clinical features

Active TB symptoms may include night sweats, fever, unexplained weight loss and tiredness. Pulmonary TB can also cause a cough, for three weeks or more, possibly with blood-streaked sputum. Any patient who has had a prolonged cough, particularly if they have had two or more courses of antibiotics, should have TB considered as a diagnosis. Consider referring your patient to their GP for investigation or directly to the TB team at your local hospital, particularly if they have been in contact with a known case or are from areas of the world with high incidence. Those who smoke, are homeless or have poor nutrition are more at risk of TB. Other vulnerable groups include people who live in overcrowded households, people with vitamin D deficiency, people in prisons and people with substance misuse issues.

Acquisition

TB is relatively difficult to contract, with close prolonged contact required. People are most likely to contract TB from their household contacts and this has implications for contact tracing. Anyone who shares a house with someone diagnosed with TB should be screened for active and latent disease. The patient should be supported to discuss their diagnosis with family and friends, in coordination with the TB nurses and multidisciplinary team. Contact tracing will be led by the TB nurse, and if there are wider contexts to be explored such as workplaces or school setting the local health protection team should also be involved to lead the contact tracing.

Diagnosis

Diagnosis of TB is made by culture and microscopy of sputum. Culture can take some time to grow, around 6–12 weeks. PCR (polymerase chain reaction) is quicker, giving a result in 1–2 days. Latent TB is diagnosed by Mantoux testing or IGRA blood tests. Latent TB can be treated to prevent active infection later in life. People who are HIV positive, in poor health, dependent on drugs or alcohol or with solid organ transplants are more at risk of progressing

from latent to active infection. Other risk factors include very young age or being elderly or immunosuppressed (Figure 68.1).

Treatment

District nurses may be involved in the administration of DOT (directly observed therapy). TB treatments range from six to twelve months. Regimes will vary according to genotyping and other clinical considerations. The patient should be supported with their nutritional requirements during treatment. Patients with infectious TB should be appropriately isolated until no longer infectious (usually until two weeks of treatment have been completed) (Figure 68.2).

Vaccination

Eligible infants should be immunised as soon as possible after birth and community healthcare professionals should do their best to facilitate this. Healthcare professionals should be aware of the most recent eligibility criteria for children and adults. More information is available from the NHS website (https://www.nhs.uk/conditions/vaccinations/bcg-tuberculosis-tb-vaccine/).

District nursing role

District nurses will understand the neighbourhood and the type of community that they are working within. The skills for the district nurse will consider how the social determinants of health affect their local area. Certain areas of the UK will have higher incidences of TB and district nurses should always be alert to the possibility of this diagnosis, particularly with latent TB infections. As a nurse not specifically working in the field of TB, they have a crucial role in making every contact count, particularly in the following:

- Ensuring prompt early diagnosis and initiation of treatment.
- Caring for patients with an early diagnosis of TB or suspected TB. The district nurse will need to do a home assessment if required to visit. The district nurse's role is to be clear about the mental and emotional state of the patient as well as their physical state following diagnosis.
- Providing treatment support for individuals with TB, liaising with all the partners in the patient's care.
- Working with underserved populations, such as the homeless, those with drug and alcohol dependency and those from high-incidence areas of the world who will be at more risk. South Asia and sub-Saharan Africa have substantially higher rates.
- Providing person-centred care. This is paramount. In many parts of the world there is significant stigma associated with TB, which may lead a patient to be fearful of their prognosis and less willing to share information due to fear of discrimination.

The team leader of the district nursing team will need to liaise with acute services, the TB nursing team and the wider multidisciplinary team and appreciate the different partners involved in the patient's care. Their role is often to lead the district nursing team in understanding the working relationship they have with acute services and primary care.

69 Prison nursing

Amanda Phillips, QN

Figure 69.1   Considerations when prescribing in prison.

Aerosols
May be used as a fire accelerant or incapacitant. Potential for inhalant abuse.

Medication in glass bottles
Glass may be broken and used as a weapon. Medication supplied in plastic containers is preferable.

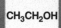

CH_3CH_2OH

Products containing alcohol
Mouthwash and ethanol based gel may be used as an intoxicant or as a base for illicit home-brew.

Figure 69.2   The reception process.

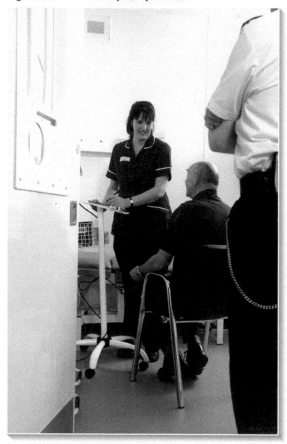

Figure 69.3   The prison environment.

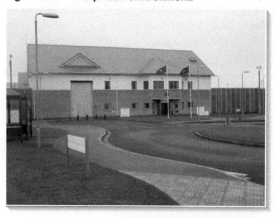

Figure 69.4   Prison nurse input.

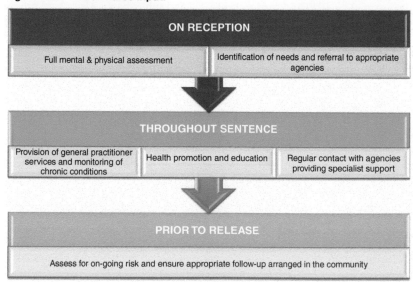

ON RECEPTION

| Full mental & physical assessment | Identification of needs and referral to appropriate agencies |

THROUGHOUT SENTENCE

| Provision of general practitioner services and monitoring of chronic conditions | Health promotion and education | Regular contact with agencies providing specialist support |

PRIOR TO RELEASE

Assess for on-going risk and ensure appropriate follow-up arranged in the community

District Nursing at a Glance, First Edition. Edited by Matthew Bradby.
© 2022 John Wiley & Sons Ltd. Published 2022 by John Wiley & Sons Ltd.

Prisons can inevitably be quite foreboding places, where the focus is on security and risk management. Healthcare facilities provided by each prison vary depending on the size of the establishment. Larger institutions provide 24-hour care with inpatient facilities and employ their own medical practitioners. Smaller prisons provide a service comparable to that of a general practice and tend to be nurse-led units providing daytime cover only.

Prison environment

Although working in a prison is inherently hazardous, the environment is designed to manage the threat of violence, with the provision of radios, alarms and CCTV cameras to minimise the risk to health practitioners.

Nursing in this setting can prove challenging, as many prisoners can have complex health requirements and at the same time the needs of the patient must be constantly weighed up against the fundamental need to maintain a safe and secure working environment. A prime example of this is the need to regulate any medication taken back to the wings (the living quarters where prisoners spend much of their time). This involves close consideration of the drug, its excipients, pharmaceutical form and the nature of the container it is stored in (Figure 69.1).

Possibly the most difficult aspect of custodial nursing is learning to deal with deceitful individuals who feign illness or symptoms in order to obtain drugs. In the prison environment, prescription drugs (particularly those capable of eliciting a psychotropic effect) are often used by detainees as a form of currency. This culture creates an ethical and professional dilemma for health practitioners, as they try to differentiate between genuine clinical need and drug-seeking behaviour. The need for sound clinical skills and a perspicacious mind is essential, therefore, if practitioners are to avoid being manipulated into providing unnecessary treatment.

In the prison environment, another significant role of the nurse is to safeguard the wellbeing of patients who may have to be forcibly restrained by prison officers. Control and restraint is a series of approved physical interventions used to manage unruly prisoners when other de-escalation techniques have proved ineffective. As a member of the healthcare team, the nurse's role is to advise prison staff of any conditions which may prove deleterious to the patient's health (such as osteoporosis, respiratory conditions or bleeding disorders) and to closely monitor the patient for signs of distress during and after the incident.

New arrivals

New prisoners are referred to as 'receptions' and are assessed by a member of the healthcare team when they first arrive. This initial assessment is a valuable tool through which the prison nurse can obtain a great deal of information about their patient's physical, mental and social history. It is also an opportunity for the practitioner to bring an air of normality to an experience which for those imprisoned for the first time is often completely alien and very intimidating (Figures 69.2 and 69.3).

The information gathered during the reception interview is used to determine the level of healthcare input that is likely to be necessary to maintain the patient's wellbeing throughout their period of incarceration. Those identified as being 'high risk' may require multidisciplinary input from substance misuse workers, mental health services or prison staff (Figure 69.4).

Mental health

A significant proportion of prisoners suffer from mental health problems, with two-thirds diagnosed with personality disorders, half suffering from depression and anxiety, and 1 in 12 diagnosed with psychosis. It is imperative that any mental health issues highlighted at the initial health assessment are addressed and managed as soon as possible. Most penal institutes utilise in-reach facilities provided by local mental health services; however, prison nurses may still have to deal with patients during crisis situations. Self-harming is commonplace amongst prisoners and nurses must be able to address both the psychological and physiological needs of the patient in these incidences.

Health promotion

A high proportion of prisoners lead unhealthy lifestyles in the period prior to their arrest that may include binge drinking, smoking and substance misuse and/or unprotected sex. Any period of imprisonment is, therefore, an ideal opportunity to interact with high-risk individuals who would not ordinarily access health promotion activities. Small changes made to a prisoner's lifestyle not only improve their health and wellbeing but also have a positive effect on the wider community into which they are released at the end of their sentence.

All prisoners are routinely offered hepatitis B immunisation and given advice on issues pertinent to their lifestyle. This may include guidance on safer injecting techniques, or highlighting the dangers of binge drinking and smoking. Prison healthcare also provides information on support services available to patients on release.

Many countries, including the UK, are dealing with an increasing number of older prisoners and some individuals may die within the prison system. Managing the healthcare needs of these individuals in a fair and safe way is a particular challenge that requires effective collaborative working with diverse professional groups and other organisations.

Prison nursing is a unique role that requires sound clinical, interpersonal and organisational skills. It involves caring for vulnerable individuals with complex health needs for whom even the smallest amount of guidance or support could prove to be the catalyst for positive change.

Nursing in defence primary healthcare

70

Katherine Moore, QN

Figure 70.1   A typical defence service hospital facility.

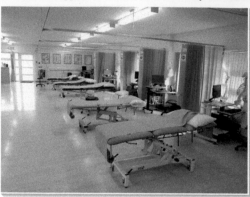

Figure 70.2   Servicewoman receiving care from nurse. Source: U.S. Army

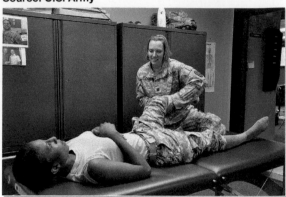

Box 70.1   Activities related to occupational health, health promotion and disease prevention.

- Smoking cessation
- Sexual health
- Contraceptive health
- Hearing conservation programme
- Spirometry
- COSSH medicals
- Travel vaccinations
- Cervical cytology
- Alcohol awareness
- Drug awareness
- Nutrition and diet advice
- Occupational medicals – aircrew, diving, gliding, medical screening, arduous training, parachute

Box 70.2   Occupational medical assessments may be needed for:

- Pilots
- Aircrew
- Air traffic controllers
- Live ammunition handlers

Medication considerations in these groups
- Sedating medication
- Analgesia
- Malaria prophylaxis
- Antidepressants
- Vaccines (anaphylaxis up to 12 hours post vaccination)

Box 70.3   Common conditions.

- Coughs and colds
- Upper respiratory tract infections
- Sprains
- Back pain
- Blisters
- Shin splints
- Microfractures
- Joints pain
- Urine infections
- Skin conditions
- Cuts and burns

Box 70.4   Deployment preparation.

- Medical fitness
  - No injuries
  - Outstanding appointments
- In date with vaccinations – offer others as appropriate
- Malaria prophylaxis
- General travel advice
- Women are not pregnant and in date with cervical cytology
- Have enough medication for duration of deployment
- No outstanding occupational requirements

Box 70.5   Vaccinations required.

National vaccination programme
- Tetanus diphtheria and inactivated polio vaccine
- Meningitis C
- MMR

Travel vaccinations
- Typhoid
- Hepatitis A
- Hepatitis B
- Yellow fever
- BCG

Risk assessment
- Meningitis ACWY
- Rabies
- Tick-borne encephalitis
- Japanese encephalitis

Biological warfare risk
- Anthrax
- Smallpox

Box 70.6   Vector-borne diseases.

- Crimean Congo haemorrhagic fever (CCHF)
- Dengue
- Japanese encephalitis
- Leishmaniasis
- Lyme disease
- Malaria
- Onchocerciasis
- Rickettsia
- Trypanosomiasis
- Yellow fever

District Nursing at a Glance, First Edition. Edited by Matthew Bradby.
© 2022 John Wiley & Sons Ltd. Published 2022 by John Wiley & Sons Ltd.

The future vision of primary healthcare is changing from being focused on the treatment of ill health to a more positive focus on the maintenance of health. This has always been the defence primary healthcare (DPHC) ethos. The role of the DPHC is to support and maintain a fit fighting force that maximises health and ensures that personnel are medically fit to meet the demands of military operations. Each service (Royal Navy, Army and RAF) serves a different purpose, which imposes different healthcare demands on medical centres (Figure 70.1). Military doctors, nurses, paramedics and medical assistants manage minor illnesses and aliments and provide medical support on all operations.

Defence primary healthcare

To maintain a fit, fighting force, ready to deploy anywhere in the world at short notice, the DPHC addresses chronic and acute health problems, minor injuries and ailments. Chronic disease management is an area of care provided to a small number of dependants and military personnel who have developed a disease whilst in service. Occupational health, health promotion and disease prevention is at the heart of care provision supplied to service personnel and their families by diverse military and civilian multidisciplinary teams (Figure 70.2 and Box 70.1). Both service and civilian military nurses need to be able to work well within diverse multidisciplinary teams in military medical centres in various environmental conditions. The main role of the civilian nurse is to provide continuity in the established workplace.

Health maintenance

It is important that service personnel are fit for their role within the military. Musculoskeletal injuries occur frequently and are managed by a multidisciplinary team of doctors, nurses and physiotherapists, as it is essential that the serviceman or woman is returned to full fitness as soon as possible. Regular health screening medicals are performed on service personnel to ensure fitness (Box 70.2). Annual medical screening is performed on specialist groups such as divers, aircrew and air traffic controllers to ensure they are fit to perform their role and to reduce the risk of adverse health events that can affect their ability.

Minor illness and ailments are common presentations at military medical centres (Box 70.3). The occupational role of service person has to be considered when treating and prescribing for minor illnesses or ailments as these can have significant effect on physical and cognitive function. Access to contraceptive and sexual health services is essential. Education, screening and treatments are available for the prevention and treatment of sexually transmitted diseases. A comprehensive contraceptive service should also be available. Referral to local NHS clinics can be made if this cannot be provided by the unit's own medical centre.

Military operations

Service personnel are deployed on military operations all over the world in diverse environmental conditions: extreme heat and cold, desert and jungle. They must be medically prepared to endure these conditions (Box 70.4). Healthcare professionals provide medical pre-deployment education for the area of deployment.

Routine travel vaccinations are administered on entering the service to ensure that the individual is protected if rapid deployment is required and so that colleagues and the local population in the operational area are protected (Box 70.5). The National Vaccination Programme is adhered to, and additional vaccinations and malaria prophylaxis are administered on risk assessment of the deployment area. Anthrax and smallpox vaccinations are offered if there is considered to be a bioterrorist risk. Many diseases are transmitted by biting arthropods (e.g. mosquitoes, flies, lice and ticks) and in many cases bite avoidance is the only means of prevention (Box 70.6). Practical bite avoidance measures should be taken to reduce risk.

It is important that individuals are at minimal risk of becoming seriously unwell on deployment. This can be a considerable burden on the operational unit and could result in the individual being aeromeded back to the UK, which could have a significant impact on the task and even the whole operation. The logistics of repatriating ill or injured military personnel back to the UK from overseas is a major task. If medical evacuation is required, specially trained medical teams are drawn from the Aeromedical Evacuation Squadron. This may require full medical support following severe injury or an escort for a condition routinely seen in primary healthcare that needs specialist treatment or referral in the UK. Aeromedical evacuation has considerable personal, administrative and financial consequences.

Families

Children of military personnel require special consideration; they are exposed to unique experiences that can include separation from a parent, who are often sent to areas of conflict, and have frequent moves and changes of schools. All of these experiences have an impact on the child. The child's ability to learn can be disrupted, they may feel isolated, find it difficult to fit in and unable to cope without support from the community, schools, school nurses and health visitors. Those children with complex educational or health needs find that the continuity of care is complicated by frequent moves.

The DPHC nurse needs to be an independent generalist who has extensive and diverse knowledge and skills that can be adapted to any situation anywhere in the world. They need to keep abreast of world affairs, and need to have a good knowledge of the geography, demography and society of countries where they may work.

71 Homeless and inclusion health nursing

Jan Keauffling, QN

Figure 71.1 Some risk factors for homelessness. Source: Webb et al. (2018), Fitzpatrick et al. (2016), Luchenski et al. (2018).

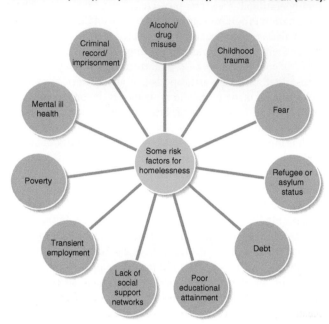

Some risk factors for homelessness

- Alcohol/drug misuse
- Childhood trauma
- Criminal record/imprisonment
- Fear
- Mental ill health
- Refugee or asylum status
- Poverty
- Debt
- Transient employment
- Poor educational attainment
- Lack of social support networks

Box 71.1 District nurse contact with people experiencing homelessness.

- Wound dressings
- Management of chronic leg ulcers
- Follow-up after hospital admission
- As part of rapid response team
- As part of integrated care team
- Palliative and end-of-life care

Box 71.2 Some issues that can impact on the person's ability to engage with healthcare.

- Previous negative experience of health services
- Problems registering with a GP due to lack of identification
- Asylum or refugee status
- Mental health issues
- Behavioural problems
- Literacy issues
- Previous missed appointments
- Attending appointments on time (no telephone, watch or alarm clock)
- Lack of transport or money for transport
- No telephone for telephone triage type services
- Intoxication
- Conflicting priorities such as need for food, drugs, alcohol, accommodation
- Zero-tolerance drug/alcohol policies
- Communication/language difficulties
- Services providing help to access healthcare may open well after all appointments at GP surgeries have already been allocated
- Fear

Box 71.3 Case study 1.

The district nurse was annoyed that she was asked to visit a patient who needed wound care at home. Why wouldn't the patient attend the Saturday wound clinic 5 miles away?

When she arrived at the address it was clear that this was bed and breakfast accommodation. Tanya was on the second floor in a cramped room, a walking frame and a wheelchair next to the bed. There was no lift in the building. She had no money for a taxi and no-one to push her the 5 miles to the clinic.

Tanya's forefoot had been amputated because of frostbite. She had been homeless for the past six months after a cycle of self-harm when her child was taken into care.

Box 71.4 Case study 2.

Jane was 35 years old when she was diagnosed with end-stage liver disease. She had been homeless for many years because of her drug and alcohol misuse and the behavioural problems that were associated with it. After her diagnosis Jane agreed to go into a hostel. She was under the care of the local palliative care team when her pain and discomfort from ascites became an issue. The district nurse came to the hostel to meet Jane along with the palliative care clinical nurse specialist and the homeless healthcare nurse. Her care plan was formulated and the district nursing team were asked to give analgesia and anti-emetics intramuscularly if oral medication failed. Jane had been worried about being able to manage her pain but hated the thought that she would be a nuisance to busy nurses who had 'really ill people to deal with'.

The district nurse called fortnightly to see Jane even if she had not needed pain relief. These visits were useful for staff at the hostel to talk through any concerns that they had and encouraged Jane to discuss her symptoms with everyone.

In the end Jane's death was sudden and unexpected. The last healthcare professional Jane had seen was the day before. The district nurse had called to give her pain relief in the middle of the night. This had been effective and she woke feeling much better. She had spent her last day with her friends and hostel staff talking, laughing and watching her beloved football team.

District Nursing at a Glance, First Edition. Edited by Matthew Bradby.
© 2022 John Wiley & Sons Ltd. Published 2022 by John Wiley & Sons Ltd.

District nurses traditionally work within the patient's home, so it might seem strange that this chapter focuses on homelessness. However, in some areas of the UK, district nurses provide all outreach healthcare for people who are homeless or living in hostels, and for the majority of nurses it will be an occasional requirement – perhaps dressing a post-operative wound for someone in bed and breakfast accommodation (Box 71.1). It is also possible that a nurse might see a sleeping bag beside the sofa of one of their usual patients, or be providing care to someone who is at risk of homelessness. Therefore the district nurse needs knowledge and skills to:

- understand the health and wellbeing needs of people experiencing homelessness and how a lack of housing might have an impact on this;
- recognise the issues that can affect and prevent the patient's engagement with health services and take steps to reduce these issues;
- recognise those at risk of homelessness and take steps to prevent it through early referral and, where appropriate, multi-agency working;
- work collaboratively with other agencies to provide high-quality end-of-life care for people in hostels and other temporary accommodation.

Homelessness

Rough sleeping is the most visible form of homelessness. However, rough sleeping is only one of four main categories of homelessness, with the other types being far less conspicuous:

- *Houselessness*: People in hostels or temporary accommodation such as women's refuges and bed and breakfasts.
- *Insecure housing*: People at risk of eviction.
- *Inadequate housing*: People in overcrowded or unfit accommodation, such as squats.

Calculation of homelessness figures is problematic, but examination of current data in the UK shows that the number of people sleeping rough and being placed in temporary accommodation is rising. Homelessness is not a fixed or permanent state and most episodes of homelessness result from a combination of personal vulnerability, limitations of social housing and inadequacies in welfare administration and support (Figure 71.1).

Impact on health

People experiencing homelessness can be affected by acute illness or long-term conditions, in the same way as the general population. Many people experiencing homelessness are likely to have multiple health problems and these can be expected to be poorly controlled with higher rates of complication. Attendance at emergency departments is higher and presentation to care is prone to be delayed to a much later stage in their illness. Hospital stays are likely to be longer because of their multiple complex health needs. In addition, high levels of smoking and poor diet amongst those experiencing homelessness can themselves lead to long-term health conditions or worsen existing health. This amalgamation of co-occurring physical ill health, mental illness and substance misuse is often referred to as trimorbidity (Box 71.2).

A lack of housing will impact on the health condition itself, but also on the ability to manage it effectively. Some examples are the following:

- Not being able to store medicines that require refrigeration or are controlled substances
- No access to kitchen equipment or appliances to improve diet
- No access to toilet facilities at night to maintain continence
- No washing facilities on the streets to keep skin and clothing clean.

Engagement and effective working

The key to health provision for people who are homeless is engagement (Box 71.3). This will not be a single consultation, but repeated attendances by people seeking healthcare. The care ordinarily provided to people who are homeless is more complex because of the lack of housing, the likelihood of trimorbidity and because health services are not planned with treatment of multiple conditions in mind. Accessing appropriate health services can therefore be difficult. Improving engagement can be achieved through improved understanding of the specific needs of homeless people and a flexibility of approach.

Although it is the case that people who are homeless are frequently perceived as unreliable and non-concordant by health workers, nurses can sometimes be viewed as uncaring by these same patients. In a study of service users experiencing homelessness, they requested that all health service providers endeavour to develop trust and acceptance, fairness and equity, with sufficient time and patience to fully engage with patients who are homeless through open, honest and supportive care. Engagement therefore requires consistent and positive relationships to be built between staff and homeless individuals, with trust and respect being key. Even with only 15 minutes to see a patient, it is vital that the interaction with nurses does not impact negatively on the homeless individual's ability to engage effectively with health services in the future (Box 71.4).

End-of-life care

A district nurse may be involved with caring for people experiencing homelessness with life-limiting illnesses in a hostel or other temporary accommodation. A primary cause of death for homeless individuals is alcohol-related liver disease. This and other diseases such as cancer, COPD and HIV require collaborative work between the hostel and a variety of specialist care staff and parallel planning. Parallel planning involves the identification of those homeless individuals who may be approaching the end of their life. Multidisciplinary support and care planning is then provided through assessment and consideration of these individuals' wishes and concerns about their ill health and its management. Although challenging, collaboration with other services to address the complex holistic needs of homeless people at the end of life is well within the capabilities of every district nurse.

The Queen's Nursing Institute operates a Homeless and Inclusion Health Programme to improve practice in this area of specialism. For more information, visit: https://www.qni.org.uk/nursing-in-the-community/homeless-health-programme/

72 Gardens, health and district nurses

Cate Wood, QN

Figure 72.1 Six steps to improved wellbeing.

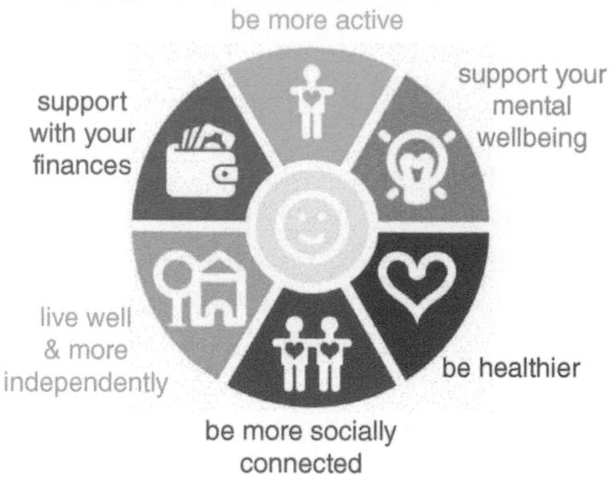

be more active

support your mental wellbeing

support with your finances

be healthier

live well & more independently

be more socially connected

Figure 72.2 Gardening, garden visiting and even images of gardens can have a positive effect on mental health.

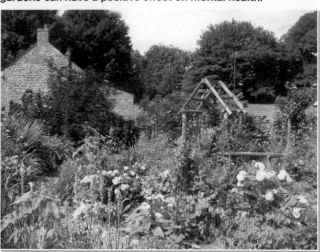

Figure 72.3 A couple opening their garden for the National Garden Scheme in aid of nursing and caring charities. Source: National Garden Scheme.

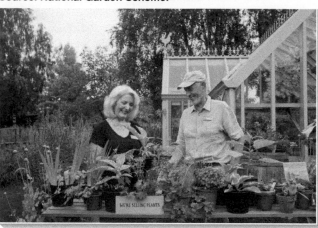

Figure 72.4 National health service social prescribing model.

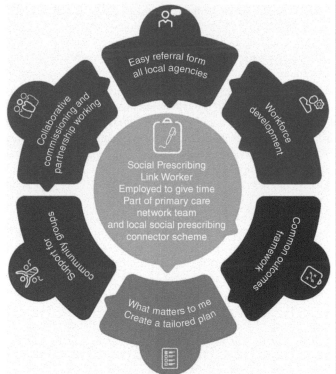

Easy referral form all local agencies

Collaborative commissioning and partnership working

Workforce development

Social Prescribing Link Worker Employed to give time Part of primary care network team and local social prescribing connector scheme

Support for community groups

Common outcomes framework

What matters to me Create a tailored plan

District Nursing at a Glance, First Edition. Edited by Matthew Bradby.
© 2022 John Wiley & Sons Ltd. Published 2022 by John Wiley & Sons Ltd.

A holistic approach to care has traditionally been the central belief of general practice in the UK. The dimensions of physical, mental and social health are each recognised as influencing overall health outcomes of patients.

Organic physical disease is often connected with psychological factors. However, recent changes in general practice, such as constraints on time, are weakening the deliverability and importance of such an approach. Human healing is more than a list of diseases and interventions. Therapeutic aids to recovery or coping with a new state of health are often found away from the traditional prescription pad. For example, gardens, gardening and being in natural environments can have positive impacts on health (Figure 72.1).

Social prescribing, sometimes known as a community referral, enables GPs, nurses and other primary care professionals to refer people to a range of local, non-clinical services. The aim of social prescribing is to improve patients' health by non-medical interventions. Long-term health problems, including stress, depression and chronic pain can benefit from social prescribing as an alternative to drugs or in addition to orthodox care. It promotes health and independence with an emphasis on prevention, patient-centred care and integration of services. Gardens and gardening are an example of social prescribing.

Outdoor spaces including gardens can reduce social isolation amongst older people and can help patients recover and manage conditions such as dementia. The Royal Horticultural Society (RHS) and the NHS joined forces at the Chelsea Flower Show in 2018 to promote the positive impact that gardening has on mental health. A 'gardening for health' forum was hosted by the Chelsea Flower Show, exploring ways to promote non-medical treatments such as gardening or enjoying green spaces.

What do gardens, health and district nursing have in common? This may sound like a conundrum, yet it is important to understand the historical connections between gardens, health and nursing. In 1859 William Rathbone, a Liverpool merchant, employed a nurse – Mary Robinson – to care for his wife in their home. Mary continued to help people in the neighbourhood after Mrs Rathbone's death. He then raised funds for the recruitment, training and employment of nurses in the deprived areas of Liverpool. This was the start of the district nursing movement, and from where the link between gardens and nursing originated.

In 1926 a fund in memory of Queen Alexandra was started to pay for nurse training and to support nurses who were retiring. Elsie Wagg (a Queen's Nursing Institute (QNI) council member), had the idea of raising money for charity through the nation's passion for gardening, by asking people to open their gardens to the public in return for a modest entry fee that would be donated to district nursing organisations affiliated with the QNI. In 1927 the National Garden Scheme was officially founded; people were invited to open their gardens and charge members of the public 'a shilling a head'; 609 gardens raised over £8000.

Since 1927 the NGS has been inviting garden owners to open their gardens to the public for charitable causes (Figures 72.2 and 72.3). In August 2017 the NGS launched their first annual 'Gardens and Health' week, dedicated to promoting the positive health impact of gardens. All the garden owners participating in this event opened their gardens free of charge for a small, private group of people who for health or social reason do not have opportunities to enjoy or visit gardens. The funds raised from opening gardens are used to benefit a number of national healthcare charities including the Queen's Nursing Institute, Macmillan Cancer Support, Marie Curie, Carers Trust, Hospice UK, Perennial, Parkinson's UK and Horatio's Garden.

The NHS has increasingly embraced social prescribing in recent years, and with the publication of the NHS Long Term Plan in 2019 this has now been formalised on a national basis, at least in England. Social prescribing link workers now act as experts in signposting people to organisations that can help promote healthier lifestyles and improve physical and mental health (Figure 72.4). It is hoped that by doing so, the burden of disease may be alleviated for individuals and long-term costs to the NHS may be better managed.

The link between gardens and health marks the spirit of the age or zeitgeist. Interests in social prescribing continue to reinvigorate holistic health practice within the rapidly changing needs and demands of primary care, placing gardens as therapy at the forefront of patient care. There is a need for robust and systematic evidence on the health benefits of green spaces, gardens and gardening to secure their place within holistic care systems as a form of social prescribing.

For more information about the National Garden Scheme visit www.ngs.org.uk.

References and further reading

References

Abdelhafiz, A.H. and Sinclair, A.J. (2013). Management of type 2 diabetes in older people. *Diabetes Therapy* 4: 13–26.

Applebaum, B. (2017). Comforting discomfort as complicity: White fragility and the pursuit of invulnerability. *Hypatia* 32(4): 862–875.

Bain, H. and Baguley, F. (2012). The management of caseloads in district nursing. *Primary Health Care* 22(4): 31–37.

Bowers, B. (2018). Evidence-based practice in community nursing. *British Journal of Community Nursing* 23(7): 336–337.

Carers UK (2014a). Care Act 2014 Key provision for carers. http://www.carersuk.org/for-professionals/policy/policy-library/care-act-2014 (accessed 19 July 2015).

Carers UK (2014b). Need to know: Transitions in and out of caring: the information challenge. http://www.carersuk.org/for-professionals/policy/policy-library/need-to-know (accessed 19 July 2015).

Carers UK (2018). State of caring 2018. https://www.carersuk.org/images/Downloads/SoC2018/State-of-Caring-report-2018.pdf (accessed 29 August 2018).

Department of Health (2010). Ready to Go? Planning the discharge and the transfer of patients from hospital and intermediate care. https://www.sheffieldmca.org.uk/UserFiles/File/Ward_Collab/Ward_Principles/Ready_to_Go_Hospital_Discharge_Planning.pdf

Department of Health (2014). Supporting the health and wellbeing of adult carers. https://www.gov.uk/government/publications/supporting-adult-carers-through-community-nursing (accessed 19 July 2015).

Department of Health and Social Care (2001). Valuing people – a new strategy for learning disability for the 21st century. https://www.gov.uk/government/publications/valuing-people-a-new-strategy-for-learning-disability-for-the-21st-century

Department of Health and Social Care (2005). National service framework: long term conditions. https://www.gov.uk/government/publications/quality-standards-for-supporting-people-with-long-term-conditions

Diabetes UK (2017). The cost of diabetes. https://www.diabetes.org.uk/resources-s3/2017-11/diabetes%20uk%20cost%20of%20diabetes%20report.pdf

Fetzer, A. and Fetzer, S. (2015). Early lipoedema diagnosis and the RCGP e-learning course. *Journal of Community Nursing, Oedema Supplement* 20(4): 6–12.

Gilburt, H. (2016). Supporting integration through new roles and working across boundaries. https://www.kingsfund.org.uk/publications/supporting-integration-new-roles-boundaries

Grundy, C. and Wheeler, H. (2018). The development of a Caseload Review tool. *British Journal of Community Nursing* 25(6): 220–226.

Guest, J.F., Ayoub, N., McIlwraith, T. et al. (2015). Health economic burden that wounds impose on the National Health Service in the UK. *BMJ Open* 5: e009283.

Hanafin, S., Roe, S., O'Dowd, M. and Barry, C. (2014). Supporting the use of evidence in community nursing: a national strategic approach. *British Journal of Community Nursing* 19(10): 496–501.

Hannan, R., Thompson, R., Worthington, A. and Rooney, P. (2013). *The Triangle of Care, Carers Included: A Guide to Best Practice for Dementia Care*. London: Carers Trust.

Hardy, G. (1981). *William Rathbone and the Early History of District Nursing: A Welfare Service, 1859–1908*. Ormskirk: Hesketh.

Haydock, D. and Evers, J. (2014). Enhancing practice teachers' knowledge and skills using collaborative action learning sets. *Community Practitioner* 87(6): 24–28.

Health Education North West (2015). Non-medical prescribing (NMP): An economic evaluation. http://www.i5health.com/NMP/NMPEconomicEvaluation.pdf (audit undertaken in 2014 and published in 2015).

International Diabetes Federation (2013). Managing older people with type 2 diabetes global guideline. https://www.idf.org/e-library/guidelines/78-global-guideline-for-managing-older-people-with-type-2-diabetes.html

Jacobs, J., Jones, E., Gabella, B. et al. (2012). Tools for implementing an evidence-based approach to public health practice. *Preventing Chronic Disease* 9: E116.

King's Fund (2016). Understanding quality in district nursing services: Learning from patients, carers and staff. https://www.kingsfund.org.uk/publications/quality-district-nursing

Knighting, K., O'Brien, M.R., Roe, B. et al. (2015). Development of the carers' alert thermometer (CAT) to identify someone struggling with caring for someone dying at home: a mixed method approach. *BMC Palliative Care* 14: 22.

Larkin, M. (2015) Developing the knowledge base about carers and personalisation: contributions made by an exploration of carers' perspectives on personal budgets and the carer-service user relationship. *Health & Social Care in the Community* 23(1):33–41.

Lee-Robichaud, H., Thomas, K., Morgan, J. and Nelson, R.L. (2010). Polyethylene glycol should be used in preference to lactulose in the treatment of chronic constipation. *Cochrane Database Systematic Reviews* (7):CD007570.

Lymphoedema UK (2014). Lipoedema UK Big Survey 2014 research report. https://www.lipoedema.co.uk/wp-content/uploads/2016/04/UK-Big-Surey-version-web.pdf

Mantzoukas, S. (2008). A review of evidence-based practice, nursing research and reflection: leveling the hierarchy. *Journal of Clinical Nursing* 17(2): 214–223.

Marmot Review (2010). Fair society, healthy lives: the Marmot Review: strategic review of health inequalities in England post-2010. https://www.gov.uk/research-for-development-outputs/fair-society-healthy-lives-the-marmot-review-strategic-review-of-health-inequalities-in-england-post-2010

Marshall, L., Bibby, J., Abbs, I (2020) Emerging evidence on COVID-19's impact on mental health and health inequalities. The Health Foundation.

Maybin, J., Charles, A. and Honeyman, M. (2016). *Understanding Quality in District Nursing Services – Learning From Patients, Carers and Staff*. London: The King's Fund.

McAndrew, S., Warren, T., Fallon, D. and Moran, P. (2012). Young, gifted and caring: A project narrative of young carers. *International Journal of Mental Health Nursing* 21:12–19.

McPherson, K.M., Kayes, N.K., Moloczij, N. and Cummins, C. (2014). Improving the interface between informal carers and formal health and social services: A qualitative study. *International Journal of Nursing Studies* 51:418–429.

MHRA (Medicines and Healthcare Regulatory Authority) (2013). Measuring blood pressure: top 10 tips. London: MHRA.

Midlands Partnership Foundation Trust (2018). Safe nurse staffing levels policy. https://www.mpft.nhs.uk/about-us/statutory-declarations/safe-staffing

District Nursing at a Glance, First Edition. Edited by Matthew Bradby.
© 2022 John Wiley & Sons Ltd. Published 2022 by John Wiley & Sons Ltd.

MIND, (2020) The Mental Health Emergency: How has the coronavirus pandemic impacted our mental health?

Morgan, P., Doherty, D., Moffatt, C. and Franks, P. (2005). The National Lymphoedema Framework Project. *Nursing Times* 101(24):48.

National Patient Safety Agency (2008). *A Risk Matrix for Risk Managers*. London: NPSA.

National Quality Board (2016). Supporting NHS providers to deliver the right staff, with the right skills, in the right place at the right time. Safe, sustainable and productive staffing. https://www.england.nhs.uk/wp-content/uploads/2013/04/nqb-guidance.pdf

National Quality Board (2018). Safe, sustainable and productive staffing: An improvement resource for the district nursing service. https://improvement.nhs.uk/documents/816/Safe_staffing_District_Nursing_final.pdf (accessed October 2020).

Nelzen, O. (2008). Prevalence of venous leg ulcer: the importance of the data collection method. *Phlebolymphology* 15(4): 143–150.

NHS (2019a). NHS Workforce race equality standard. https://www.england.nhs.uk/about/equality/equality-hub/equality-standard/

NHS (2019b). The eatwell guide. https://www.nhs.uk/live-well/eat-well/the-eatwell-guide/ (accessed October 2020).

NHS (2020). Friends and family test. https://www.nhs.uk/using-the-nhs/about-the-nhs/friends-and-family-test-fft/

NHS Digital (2017). Health and care of people with learning disabilities standardised mortality ratio indicator. https://digital.nhs.uk/data-and-information/publications/statistical/health-and-care-of-people-with-learning-disabilities/standardised-mortality-ratio-indicator

NHS England (2017). Improving through inclusion. https://www.england.nhs.uk/wp-content/uploads/2017/08/inclusion-report-aug-2017.pdf

NHS England (2020). Releasing time to care. https://www.england.nhs.uk/improvement-hub/productives/

NHSE/QNI (2014). Developing a national district nurse workforce planning framework. https://www.qni.org.uk/wp-content/uploads/2016/09/district_nursing_workforce_planning_report.pdf

NICE (National Institute for Health Care Excellence) (2014). Constipation in children and young people. Quality standard [QS62]. https://www.nice.org.uk/guidance/qs62/chapter/List-of-quality-statements

NICE (National Institute for Health Care Excellence) (2017). NICE guideline [NG51] Updated 13 September 2017. Sepsis: recognition, diagnosis and early management. https://www.nice.org.uk/guidance/NG51/chapter/Recommendations#identifying-people-with-suspected-sepsis

NICE (National Institute for Health Care Excellence) (2018). NICE guideline [NG115]. Chronic obstructive pulmonary disease in over 16s: diagnosis and management. https://www.nice.org.uk/guidance/ng115

Nursing and Midwifery Council (2016). The code: Professional standards of practice and behaviour for nurses, midwives and nursing associates. https://www.nmc.org.uk/standards/code/

Nursing and Midwifery Council (2018a). Standards for pre-registration nursing programmes: Part 3 of Realising professionalism: Standards for education and training. https://www.nmc.org.uk/standards/standards-for-nurses/standards-for-pre-registration-nursing-programmes/

Nursing and Midwifery Council (2018b). Part 2: Standards for student supervision and assessment. https://www.nmc.org.uk/globalassets/sitedocuments/standards-of-proficiency/standards-for-student-supervision-and-assessment/student-supervision-assessment.pdf

Nursing and Midwifery Council (2018c). Future nurse: Standards of proficiency for registered nurses. https://www.nmc.org.uk/globalassets/sitedocuments/education-standards/future-nurse-proficiencies.pdf

Pedler, M. and Abbott, C. (2008). Am I doing it right? Facilitating action learning for service improvement. *Leadership in Health Services* 21(3): 185–199.

Queen's Nursing Institute (2014). 2020 vision: five years on. https://www.qni.org.uk/resources/2020-vision-five-years/

Queen's Nursing Institute (2016). Understanding safe caseloads in the district nursing service. https://www.qni.org.uk/wp-content/uploads/2017/02/Understanding_Safe_Caseloads_in_District_Nursing_Service_V1.0.pdf

Queen's Nursing Institute (2018). Nursing in the digital age: using technology to support patients in the home. https://www.qni.org.uk/resources/nursing-in-the-digital-age/

Quickfall, J. (2004). Developing a model for culturally competent primary care nursing for asylum applicants and refugees in Scotland: a review of the literature. *Diversity in Health and Social Care* 1(1): 53–64.

Raelin, J.A. (1998). Work-based learning in practice. *Journal of Workplace Learning* 10(6/7): 280–283.

Rennard, S.I. and Calverley, P. (2003). Rescue! Therapy and the paradox of the Barcalounger. *European Respiratory Journal* 21: 916–917.

Rodger, D., Neill, M.O. and Nugent, L. (2015). Informal carers' experiences of caring for older adults at home: a phenomenological study. *British Journal of Community Nursing* 15(20):6 280–285.

Schofield, J.K., Fleming, D., Grindlay, D. and Williams, H. (2011). Skin conditions are the commonest new reason people present to general practitioners in England and Wales. *British Journal of Dermatology* 165(5): 1044–1050.

The Health Foundation (1995). About the Francis Inquiry. https://www.health.org.uk/about-the-francis-inquiry

Thompson, C., McCaughan, D., Cullum, N. et al. (2005). Barriers to evidence-based practice care nursing – why viewing decision-making as context is helpful. *Journal of Advanced Nursing* 52(4): 432–444.

O'Shea N., (2021) Covid-19 and the nation's mental health: May 2021. Centre for Mental Health. https://www.centreformentalhealth.org.uk/publications/covid-19-and-nations-mental-health-may-2021

World Health Organization (2003). Adherence to long-term therapies. https://www.who.int/chp/knowledge/publications/adherence_full_report.pdf

World Health Organization (2018). Palliative care. https://www.who.int/news-room/facts-in-pictures/detail/palliative-care

Further reading

General

Calverley, P., Pauwels, R., Dagger, R. et al. (2005). Relationship between respiratory symptoms and medical treatment in exacerbations of COPD. *European Respiratory Journal* 26(3): 406–413.

Cancer Research UK (2020). Cancer statistics for the UK. https://www.cancerresearchuk.org/health-professional/cancer-statistics-for-the-uk

Chilton, S. and Bain, H. (2017). *A Textbook of Community Nursing*. London: Routledge.

Cohen, S. (2018). *The District Nurse, a Pictorial History*. Barnsley: Pen & Sword History.

Cooper, G. (2010). Early diagnosis of lymphoedema helps to reduce its psychological and social impact. *Nursing Times* 106(49/50): 15–17.

International Lymphoedema Framework. *International Consensus: Best Practice for the Management of Lymphoedema*. London: MEP Ltd, 2006.

King's Fund (2016). Understanding quality in district nursing services. https://www.kingsfund.org.uk/publications/quality-district-nursing

Lipoedema UK. *Booklet for Women and Professionals to Understand the Condition of Lipoedema*. Copies available from info@lipoedema.co.uk, quoting BJCNLUKW@HCP002

Moffat, C.J., Franks, P.J., Doherty, D.C. et al. (2003). Lymphoedema, an underestimated health problem. *Quarterly Journal of Medicine* 96(10): 731–738.

National Quality Board (2018). Safe, sustainable and productive staffing – an improvement resource for the district nursing service. https://improvement.nhs.uk/documents/816/Safe_staffing_District_Nursing_final.pdf

O'Brien, L. (2012). *District Nursing Manual of Clinical Procedures*. Chichester: John Wiley & Sons.

Queen's Nursing Institute (2019). International community nursing observatory. https://www.qni.org.uk/explore-qni/icno/

Queen's Nursing Institute and Royal College of Nursing (2019). Outstanding models of district nursing report. https://www.qni.org.uk/resources/outstanding-models-of-district-nursing-report/

RCGP Training. *Lipoedema – An Adipose Tissue Disorder*. Online course free to all healthcare professionals. The Royal College of Practitioners. https://elearning.rcgp.org.uk/course/search.php?search=Adipose+tissue+disorder

Sines, D., Aldridge-Bent, S., Fanning, A. et al. (2013). *Community and Public Health Nursing*, 5th Ed. Chichester: John Wiley & Sons.

COVID-19 care

National Institute for Health and Care Excellence (2020). COVID-19 rapid guideline: managing symptoms (including at the end of life) in the community [NG163], 3 April 2020. https://www.nice.org.uk/guidance/ng163/resources/covid19-rapid-guideline-managing-symptoms-including-at-the-end-of-life-in-the-community-pdf-66141899069893

Queen's Nursing Institute (2020). Coronavirus information centre. https://www.qni.org.uk/nursing-in-the-community/care-home-nurses-network/coronavirus-information-centre/

Evidence-based practice

Goodorally, V. (2014). Developing and implementing a culturally and ethnically sensitive family assessment tool for people living with dementia and their families. https://www.fons.org/library/report-details/55736

Mathieson, A., Grande, G. and Luker, K. (2019). Strategies, facilitators and barriers to implementation of evidence-based practice in community nursing: a systematic mixed-studies review and qualitative synthesis. *Primary Health Care Research & Development* 20: e6.

Mulloy, D.F. and Hughes, R.G. (2008). Wrong-site surgery: A preventable medical error. Ch 36 in *Patient Safety and Quality: An Evidence-Based Handbook for Nurses* (ed. Hughes, R.G.). Rockville, MD: Agency for Healthcare Research and Quality.

Detection and management of frailty

Faller, J.W., Pereira, D.D.N., De Souza, S. et al. (2019). Instruments for the detection of frailty syndrome in older adults: A systematic review. *PLOS One* 14: e0216166.

Fried, L.P., Tangen, C.M., Walston, J. et al. (2001). Cardiovascular health study collaborative research group. Frailty in older adults: evidence for a phenotype. *Journal of Gerontology Series A Biological Sciences and Medical Sciences* 56.

Rockwood, K., Hogan, D.B. and Macknight, C. (2000). Conceptualisation and measurement of frailty in elderly people. *Drugs & Aging* 17: 295–302.

Turner, G. and Clegg, A. (2014). Best practice guidelines for the management of frailty: A British Geriatrics Society, Age UK and Royal College of General Practitioners report. *Age and Ageing* 43.

Community palliative care

Royal College of General Practice and Marie Curie UK (2019). The Daffodil Standards: General practice standards for advanced serious illness and end of life care. https://www.rcgp.org.uk/daffodilstandards

National Institute for Health and Care Excellence (2015). Care of dying adults in the last days of life [NG31]. 16 December 2015. https://www.nice.org.uk/guidance/ng31/resources/care-of-dying-adults-in-the-last-days-of-life-pdf-1837387324357

End-of-life anticipatory prescribing

Bowers, B., Ryan, R., Kuhn, I. and Barclay, S. (2019). Anticipatory prescribing of injectable medications for adults at the end of life in the community: A systematic literature review and narrative synthesis. *Palliative Medicine* 33(2): 160–177.

Wilson, E., Morbey, H., Brown, J., et al. (2015). Administering anticipatory medications in end-of-life care: a qualitative study of nursing practice in the community and in nursing homes. *Palliative Medicine* 29(1): 60–70.

Advanced end-of-life decision-making

National Council for Palliative Care/NHS National End of Life Care Programme (2013). Advanced decisions to refuse treatment: A guide for health and social care professionals. https://www.england.nhs.uk/improvement-hub/wp-content/uploads/sites/44/2017/11/Advance-Decisions-to-Refuse-Treatment-Guide.pdf

ReSPECT (2017). What is ReSPECT? https://learning.respectprocess.org.uk/wp-content/uploads/2017/06/What-is-ReSPECT-download.pdf

Resuscitation Council UK (2020). ReSPECT. https://www.resus.org.uk/respect

Grief and bereavement care

Corr, C.A. (2019) The 'five stages' in coping with dying and bereavement: strengths, weaknesses and some alternatives. *Mortality* 24(4): 405–417.

Cruse Bereavement Care (2020). Coping with grief. https://www.cruse.org.uk/get-help/coping-grief

eMentalHealth.ca (2017). Grief and bereavement: information for primary care. https://www.ementalhealth.ca/Canada/Grief-and-Bereavement/index.php?m=article&ID=18641

Hall, C. (2014). Bereavement theory: recent developments in our understanding of grief and bereavement. *Bereavement Care* 33(1): 7–12.

Index

District Nursing at a Glance, First Edition. Edited by Matthew Bradby.
© 2022 John Wiley & Sons Ltd. Published 2022 by John Wiley & Sons Ltd.